Endorsem

"This is a gem of a book. Clearly writt[...], [...] sustains an easy and informative approach in terms that can be well understood by those for whom it is intended, the many women and men from all walks of life who stand at risk of serious heart disease. And this is done without oversimplification or loss of accuracy. A consistent theme is that of prevention with sensible, practical, and effective recommendations for a heart-healthy lifestyle.

"All Americans should read this book, not only to learn more about themselves as marvelously complex living beings, but especially *to learn how easy it could be* to significantly reduce the immense burden of heart disease that is borne by modern society. Dr. Sauvage and his team should be complimented on this carefully crafted, clear, and articulate account of the greatest threat to human health we face today in the United States, and what steps we should take to control it."

- **David M. Robinson, PhD**
Deputy Director, Heart and Vascular Diseases
National Heart, Lung, and Blood Institute
National Institutes of Health, Bethesda, Maryland

"In *You Can Beat Heart Disease,* Dr. Lester Sauvage, a renowned cardiovascular surgeon, describes in *simple, everyday language* what the cardiovascular system is and how it works and relates to the rest of the body. Moreover, he clearly explains the disease process, hardening of the arteries, which can cause the breakdown of this vital system, the major cause of death in the United States. But above all, *You Can Beat Heart Disease* is a message of hope clearly pointing out successful treatment options for patients with cardiovascular disease while emphasizing a simple, step-by-step program for the prevention of this scourge of modern civilization. Dr. Sauvage has produced a *real gem."*

- **John A. Mannick, MD**
Mosely Distinguished Professor of Surgery
Harvard Medical School, Boston, Massachusetts

i

"This *concise book* addresses the risk factors associated with the development of heart and artery diseases and provides a detailed approach that will help you keep well. *You Can Beat Heart Disease* is important for potential patients (nearly everyone), actual patients, and physicians alike."

- Thomas J. Fogarty, MD
Professor of Surgery
Division of Vascular Surgery
Stanford University School of Medicine, Stanford, California

"*You Can Beat Heart Disease* gives the reader a step-by-step, highly *effective plan* for combating the *deadliest disease* in the industrialized world. If keeping your heart healthy concerns you, consider adding this authoritative, clearly written, and easily understood guide to your personal library."

- Denton A. Cooley, MD
President and Surgeon-in-Chief
Texas Heart Institute, Houston, Texas

"Dr. Sauvage has prepared the *most comprehensive yet understandable book for* the education of *patients* with vascular disease *that I have ever seen.* It contains a wealth of information that is beautifully illustrated and presented with the upbeat, common-sense approach for which he is so well known. Because of this book, Dr. Sauvage will attain the *fondest hope of every medical author* -- that is, to help patients he will never meet, in places he will never visit."

- Norman R. Hertzer, MD
Chairman, Department of Vascular Surgery
The Cleveland Clinic Foundation, Cleveland, Ohio

"Just take 70 seconds and read the five cardinal rules for heart-healthy living (pages 192-194) and add five to ten high quality years to your life. *What a bargain!*"

- Peter Gloviczki, MD
Professor of Surgery
Division of Vascular Surgery, Mayo Clinic, Rochester, Minnesota

"Heart and other arterial diseases kill nearly one out of every two American women -- yet this disease remains shrouded in confusion. Dr. Sauvage has performed a true feat by writing a *straight-forward, understandable book* that dispels much of the confusion and, because of this, will *save many lives*. Reading this *book is a must* for both heart patients and the general public."

- **Nancy L. Snyderman, MD**
Medical Correspondent, ABC News
New York, New York

"*This is a remarkable book.* Though written for laymen, a physician may take rewarding interest in reading it, too. It will help him brush up on his communication skills with his patients.

"The book describes in flowing and lively language *understandable* to any intelligent, non-medical reader the anatomy, physiology, pathology, and therapeutics of the diseases of the heart and arteries. *There is not a question I can think of that a patient might ask for which this book does not provide an answer.*

"Two features struck me as particularly noteworthy. First, there is a profusion of simple but accurate line drawings to illustrate every detail suitable for pictorial representation. Perhaps even more impressively, the last chapter is a seldom seen, extraordinary summary of the spiritual values of what used to be called the art of healing. In this cynical modern world, putting such sentiments on paper is an act of great moral courage. The last lines reprint the *Prayer of St. Francis,* perhaps the tenderest summation of what human goodness is."

- **D. Emerick Szilagyi, MD**
Chairman Emeritus, Department of Surgery, Henry Ford Hospital, Detroit
Professor of Surgery Emeritus, University of Michigan School of Medicine
Founding Editor, *Journal of Vascular Surgery*

"Dr. Lester Sauvage is one of the pioneers of heart surgery. Yet he is more than a pioneering surgeon; he is a *visionary physician* who addresses not only the causes and prevention of heart disease, but also the soul of his patients."

- Dean Ornish, MD
Author, *Dean Ornish's Program for Reversing Heart Disease*
President & Director, Preventive Medicine Research Institute
Clinical Professor of Medicine
School of Medicine, University of California, San Francisco

"Upon opening this book you will be more than surprised. In a pocket-sized volume of some 300 pages you will find virtually *everything you need to know* about heart-healthy living, the background of modern cardiology, and the prevention and treatment of cardiovascular disease. And there's more. This fund of information is presented in such a clear manner that even the most inexperienced and unsophisticated reader can understand it.

"Almost every page is specifically and instructively illustrated, and every topic is simply and concisely described. As I thumbed through this book before settling back to read it carefully, I wondered whether Dr. Sauvage would get to the subject of stents, or pacemakers, or a glossary, but no sooner had these ideas occurred to me than I came across these very subjects. And even more.

"Dr. Sauvage's extraordinary devotion to people shines through every page, exemplified by his citing of the Prayer of St. Francis which clearly enunciates his personal beliefs. Goodness of spirit shines forth like nothing I have seen before. I am not given to hyperbole, at least not easily, but in this case I can say that it is the *best book of its kind that I have ever read,* and I will cherish ownership of the final edition once it's in my hands."

- Victor Parsonnet, MD
Director of Surgical Research, Newark Beth Israel Medical Center
Clinical Professor of Surgery
New Jersey College of Medicine & Dentistry

Endorsements continued on pages 300-310.

iv

You Can Beat Heart Disease: How to Defeat America's # 1 Killer "Third Edition"

Medical Disclaimer: The author, editors, and publisher have made all reasonable efforts to ensure the accuracy and completeness of the information contained in this book. Health care is dynamic, and new research may be expected to add knowledge which may change future clinical recommendations. The author, editors, and publisher disclaim any liability or responsibility for injury or damage to persons or property which is incurred, directly or indirectly, as a consequence of the use and application of any of the contents of this book. It is the reader's responsibility to know and follow local care instructions provided by health care professionals with specific knowledge of the particular reader's own circumstances.

Publisher's Cataloging-in-Publication Data
(Provided by Quality Books, Inc.)

Sauvage, Lester R., 1926-
    You can beat heart disease : how to defeat America's #1 killer/ Lester R. Sauvage ; with Carol P. Garzona, prevention consultant ; Kathryn D. Barker , and Warren A. Berry, illustrators
    p. cm.
    Includes index
    Preassigned LCCN: 99-76689
    ISBN 0-9663788-5-7

    1. Heart--Diseases--Prevention.   2. Heart--Diseases--Treatment.   3. Atherosclerosis
    I. Title

    RC681.S28 2000   616.12
                        QBI00-24

YOU CAN BEAT HEART DISEASE

How to Defeat America's # 1 Killer

LESTER R. SAUVAGE, MD

with
Carol P. Garzona, Prevention Consultant,
Kathryn D. Barker, Medical Artist and Calligrapher,
and
Warren A. Berry, Director of Computer Graphics
& Medical Photography

THE HOPE HEART INSTITUTE

Better Life Press, LLC
Seattle, Washington

TABLE OF CONTENTS

Foreword by Jerry Goldstone, MD x
Prevention: Cornerstone of Good Health xiv
Acknowledgments xvi

Primary Strategy to Beat Heart Disease 1

Section I: **The Human Body**: Its Systems and
Its Greatest Killers -- Hardening
of the Arteries (Atherosclerosis)
and Clot Formation 2-83

Section II: **Diagnosis** of the Two Main
Complications of Atherosclerosis 84-111

• General Considerations 85-87
• Blockage 88-107
• Aneurysm Formation 108-111

Section III: **Prevention** of Atherosclerosis
and Its Complications by
How We Live Our Lives 112-189

• Introduction 113-115
• Smoking -- *Deadly Foe* 116-135
• **Better Life Diet***-- *True Friend* 136-160

Introduction 136
Nutritional Basis* 137-152
Meal Plan ** 153-160

• Exercise -- *Essential Ally of Diet* .. 161-187
• Stress -- *Potential Killer* 188-189

* with Robert H. Knopp, MD
** by Anna Martin, BS, and Evette Hackman, PhD, RD

Section IV: **A Simple Nonsurgical Plan**
for a Long and Youthful Life 190-199

• General Considerations 191-192
• Five Cardinal Rules............................ 192-195
• Three Additional Strategies........... 196-199

Section V: **Surgical Procedures**
for Arteries Irreversibly Damaged
by Atherosclerosis and
Its Complications: 200-249

• Two Types of Operations:
  Vascular and Endovascular............ 202-211
• Surgery to Increase Blood Supply
  to the Heart 212-227
  to the Brain 228-229
  to the Kidneys 230-232
  to the Legs 233-247
• Surgery for Aortic Aneurysms
  thoracic 248
  abdominal 249

Section VI: **Related Heart Topics**................................ 250-266

• Pacemaking and conducting
  systems of the Heart...................... 251-253
• Artificial pacemakers for the Heart 254-257
• Cardiopulmonary resuscitation
  (CPR) 258-260
• Automatic internal cardiac
  defibrillator (AICD) 261-263
• Heart transplantation 264-266

Table of Contents

Section VII: Spiritual Reflections 267-270

Section VIII: Glossary * 271-290

Review Questions 291-293

About the Author and Team Members 294-295

Message from Better Life Press 296

Need for Research 297-299

Endorsements (Completion) 300-310

Concluding Thoughts 311

Index 312-316

* **This is not the usual glossary consisting of definitions. It is instead an easily understood series of mini-lectures of key subjects. Browsing through them first will assist you in making the reading of this book a powerful means to attain a long and youthful life.**

Foreword
by
Jerry Goldstone, MD

Professor of Surgery
Case Western Reserve University
School of Medicine
Chief, Division of Vascular Surgery
University Hospitals of Cleveland
Cleveland, Ohio

This book is *about* each and every one of us, and it's *for* each and every one of us.

It's a book about our hearts and blood vessels that examines the wonders of our anatomy, physiology, biochemistry, biophysics -- and yes, even, spirituality.

No scientist or engineer could imagine being able to design, let alone build, so complex a pumping, distribution, and exchange system that could possibly work as efficiently and effectively as our cardiovascular system.

Most amazing of all, this system is expected to work flawlessly, without rest, for 80 to 100 years or more -- even when it's severely and repeatedly abused.

But like all complex systems, breakdowns and failures are inevitable, and as Dr. Sauvage and his team point out, cardiovascular disease is the leading cause of death in the United States, causing more deaths than cancer, accidents, and infections combined. Thus, it behooves us to learn more about cardiovascular disease so that its warning signs can be recognized and dealt with in order to prevent disability and death due to heart attacks, sudden stoppage of the heart, congestive heart failure, strokes, obesity, diabetes, blindness, kidney failure, decreased walking capacity, limb loss, and hemorrhage from ruptured aneuryms.

Another important reason to learn about the cardiovascular system is that dealing with diseases of the heart and blood vessels often requires choices to be made among and between various diagnostic tests, pharmaceutical agents, surgical procedures, and lifestyle changes. I believe it is important for each affected person to play an important role in making these choices. Fortunately, long gone are the days when physicians told patients "This is what you need," and the patients faithfully responded, "Yes sir, you're the doctor."

Now, the choice is largely the patient's, while the physician's role is to provide information in order to help the patient make that choice. Unfortunately, more information is frequently needed or desired than many physician-patient consultations provide.

That is why this book, *You Can Beat Heart Disease*, is so important. It explains in clear and easily understandable words, illustrations, and x-rays what the cardiovascular system does, how it is made, how it works, what happens when it becomes diseased and doesn't work, and what can be done to fix it.

The book is based largely on the life-long experience of Dr. Lester Sauvage, a noted cardiovascular surgeon and research director, who spent 33 years repairing the hearts and blood vessels of thousands of grateful patients. What better way is there to gain understanding of the human cardiovascular system than to reconstruct it day in and day out? Who better understands the working of a Ferrari than a veteran Ferrari mechanic?

In spite of the fact that Dr. Sauvage is a surgeon, not all of the therapeutic options discussed in this book involve the traditional surgical maneuvers of cutting and sewing. The new, minimally invasive, catheter-based techniques are also appropriately described and discussed. Often the choice is between no operation or procedure, a catheter-based procedure, and a standard major operation. Aided by their doctors, well-informed patients are able to make these important decisions.

There is another lesson, perhaps even more important, that we will learn from this book. This lesson is that cardiovascular disease can be minimized and, in many cases, prevented by taking care of our bodies and minds by avoiding the things that we already know damage the heart and blood vessels: **smoking, eating the wrong foods, not exercising, accumulating excess weight, and being under damaging stress.** We should also be doing more of the things that we know will lower our cardiovascular disease risk, such as following Dr. Sauvage's Better Life Diet©, exercising regularly, and taking anti-oxidant and anti-platelet medications.

The preventive strategies Dr. Sauvage wishes all of us to implement are consistent with the well-known adage that an ounce of prevention is worth a pound of cure.

No health care system can treat and cure every illness. And this is where the responsibility clearly falls on the shoulders of each and every one of us. As individuals, and collectively as a society, it is up to each of us to take care of our own cardiovascular system, and we need to begin doing so at a young age to enable this complex system to run smoothly into old age at low medical cost.

Dr. Sauvage and his team have done us all a great service by providing so much valuable information in such a concise form. Now it's up to us to put this information to good use.

Jerry Goldstone, MD

Prevention

Cornerstone of Good Health
at
An Affordable Cost

This book, *You Can Beat Heart Disease*, emphasizes that prevention is the cornerstone upon which we build our defense against the Western world's #1 killer, heart disease. For those who develop the complications of hardened arteries (pp. 77-83, blockages and ballooned-out walls), either because they followed no prevention program, started their program too late, or followed an inadequate program, surgical procedures can still come to the rescue. But such "last-minute heroics" should not be our primary objective. Instead, let's make prevention our goal. For best results, patients who **must undergo an operation** have a critical need to combine the best of surgery (pp 200-249) with the best of prevention (pp. 112-199) for the rest of their lives.

In *You Can Beat Heart Disease*, we bring you vital medical information, including the *Better Life Diet and Exercise Program*, which can help you defeat the deadly arterial diseases of the heart, brain, kidneys, other organs, and extremities. Prevention can eliminate the need for operations in many people. For those who require surgery, preventive strategies must become an integral part of their aftercare in order to avoid having new blockages and ballooned-out walls develop in the future.

Following the five cardinal rules for heart healthy (fit) living (pp. 192-194) will help you live a long, healthy, and happy life. Indeed, prevention is the cornerstone of this program. You will find this strategic plan to be sensible, effective, and enjoyable. The only requirement for success is your personal commitment.

After reading this book, you will have a broader working knowledge of how your body functions. This information base will enable you to protect the inner walls of your arteries from becoming hardened and having clots form on their flow surfaces. **Hardened arteries and clots** cause heart attacks, sudden cardiac death, congestive heart failure, strokes, high blood pressure, kidney failure, limb loss, and aneurysm rupture. These conditions kill more people than cancer, accidents, and infections combined.

Learning how to prevent heart disease is even more important than learning how to treat it. Since how we live largely determines whether our arteries will remain healthy, we emphasize the individual's essential role in maintaining or regaining heart health. This book will show you how to do this.

There is another reason why *prevention* is important -- the rising cost of health care. The harsh economic reality is that our retired population is increasing rapidly and demanding high-tech care. This could mean bankruptcy for Medicare early in this century. It's simple arithmetic. Far more people are receiving benefits today than 30 years ago. The tax base can no longer keep up. Something has to give - - - and soon.

For the Medicare and Medicaid systems of the United States to remain solvent as greater numbers of our citizens live longer, we must lower the total medical cost of keeping our older citizens healthy. *Each* of us has a responsibility to ourselves, our children, and our nation to make the lifestyle choices that will help us live as healthily as possible. Making the appropriate choices for good health is, in fact, an obligation of responsible citizenship.

Our national goal must be to give the best care to all who need it. But for this to be economically feasible, we must **decrease the number who require costly treatment.** We ask all who read this book to make the lifestyle choices that will help makes this goal become a reality and to encourage others to do the same. By working together we can succeed in this vital cause.

xv

ACKNOWLEDGMENTS

I am deeply grateful to the following people for their invaluable contributions that have made this book possible:

My staff at The Hope Heart Institute -- **Eli Chiaviello** and **Carol Alto, BA,** for their essential assistance in so many critical ways, both ordinary and complex.

Mary Ann Harvey, MA, Medical Editor of The Hope Heart Institute, for editorial and grammatical guidance.

Josh Rosenfeld of the Institute's Department of Clinical Research for verifying the incredible facts about our amazing bodies that are in this book.

Jeffrey D. Robinson, MD, and **Philip J. Vogelzand, MD,** of the Department of Radiology of the Providence Seattle Medical Center for advice on radiologic matters.

Peter A. Demopulos, MD; Milton T. English, MD; Bert Green, MD; C. Gordon Hale, MD; Tom R. Hornsten, MD; Peter B. Mansfield, MD; Michael Martin, MD; Gary E. Oppenheim, MD; and **David C. Warth, MD;** of the Providence Seattle Heart Center for up-to-date details of current cardiology and endovascular coronary surgery.

Kai Johansen, MD, PhD, and **Michael Zammit, MD,** of the Providence Seattle Vascular Center for up-to-date details of peripheral vascular surgery.

Thomas H. DeBuys, JD, -- lawyer, friend, heart patient of Donald W. Miller Jr., MD, and Peter A. Demopulos, MD, and probing student of the body's lipid chemistry -- for manuscript editing and sharing his rich knowledge with me.

Reneé Belfor,RD, Susie Wang, RD, and **Alison Evert, RD,** of the Nutrition Department of the Providence Seattle Medical Center for advice on dietary matters.

Robert H. Knopp, MD, for working with me in designing the Better Life Diet©.

Anna Martin, BS, and **Evette Hackman, PhD, RD,** for creating a seven day meal plan for, and nutritional analysis of, the **Better Life Diet**©.

Keith Fujioka, BS, RVT, President/CEO Pacific Vascular, Inc., and his staff of the Pacific Vascular Laboratory at the Providence Seattle Medical Center for assistance on ultrasound matters.

Dick Delson for manuscript editing.

Stan Emert, JD, for critical work at every level in all phases of this project, including developing effective plans to bring this book and its companions, *The Better Life Diet* and *The Open Heart,* to the widest possible audiences.

Arthur Nakata for designing a cover that precisely captures the spirit of this book.

My family for their devoted support and encouragement throughout this joyful endeavor, **especially my dear wife, Mary Ann,** for her invaluable advice concerning all aspects of this project and to our **son, John,** for his essential help in making this book reader-friendly.

To **Jerry Goldstone, MD**, for writing the Foreword and to the many others who have endorsed this book, I am deeply grateful. They are:

Wiley F. Barker, MD

John J. Bergan, MD

Bradford C. Berk, MD, PhD

Nicholas J. Bez

Denton A. Cooley, MD

Herbert Dardik, MD

R. Clement Darling III, MD

Mr. Aires A.B. Barros D'Sa, MD

Calvin B. Ernst, MD

Thomas J. Fogarty, MD

Julie Ann Freischlag, MD

Peter Gloviczki, MD

H. Leon Greene, MD

Howard P. Greisler, MD

C. Rollins Hanlon, MD

Norman R. Hertzer, MD

Glenn C. Hunter, MD

Anthony M. Imparato, MD

Kaj H. Johansen, MD, PhD

J. Ward Kennedy, MD

John F. (Jack) Kiley

John W. Kirklin, MD

Robert L. Kistner, MD

Robert H. Knopp, MD

Floyd D. Loop, MD

John A. Mannick, MD

S. A. Mellick, CBE, MD

Yasutsugu Nakagawa, MD

Lloyd M. Nyhus, MD

John L. Ochsner, MD

Dean Ornish, MD

Victor Parsonnet, MD

Malay Patel, MD

Malcolm O. Perry, MD

Joseph C. Piscatella

Charles G. Rob, MD

Francis Robicsek, MD, PhD

David M. Robinson, PhD

Robert B. Rutherford, MD

Stephen M. Schwartz, MD, PhD

Nancy L. Snyderman, MD

Ronald J. Stoney, MD

D. Emerick Szilagyi, MD

Jesse E. Thompson, MD

Frank J. Veith, MD

J. Leonel Villavicencio, MD

Vallee L. Willman, MD

James S.T. Yao, MD, PhD

Christopher K. Zarins, MD

SPECIAL ACKNOWLEDGMENT

For 33 years of my life, I had the good fortune to conduct my surgical practice at the *Providence Seattle Medical Center.* From that experience, I came to deeply appreciate the tremendous value of kind and loving care administered in an atmosphere of scientific excellence.

It is easy for the human touch to be lost in the hurried, high-tech, impersonal medical practice of today. Yet, the care provided by the dedicated nursing staff at Providence showed concern for all - - including the poor and the vulnerable.

Though change is part of life, fundamental values must endure if we are to truly advance. Two years ago (2000), the *Providence* and *Swedish Medical Centers* of Seattle merged and now continue their traditions of excellence together.

Primary Strategy
to
Beat Heart Disease

In this book we present

general **concepts**,

specific **information**,

and clear **directions**

to help you defeat heart disease

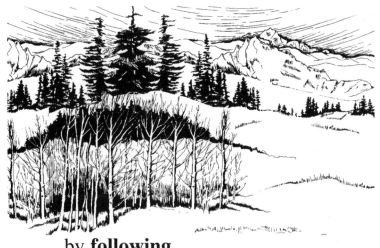

by **following**

the **five cardinal rules** for

heart-healthy (fit) living.

Section I:

The Human Body

Its Systems and Its
Greatest Killers -- Hardening
of the Arteries (Atherosclerosis)
and Clot Formation

Introduction 4-7
The Cell 8-11
The Life Cycle 12-15

The 11 Major Body Systems 16-39

1. Musculoskeletal System 18
2. Nervous System 19
3. Cardiovascular System,
   an Overview 20-21
4. Hematopoietic (Blood Cell
   Forming) System 22-23
5. Lymphatic/Immune System 24-25
6. Respiratory System 26-27
7. Digestive System 28-29
8. Urinary System 30-33
9. Endocrine System 34-35
10. Reproductive System 36-37
11. Integumentary (Skin) System 38-39

Boundary Organ Concept 40-43

The Cardiovascular System, a Detailed Examination of Its Three Main Parts 44-67

   1. *Power Source*, the Heart 45-55

      • Circulatory Cycle and
        Color Changes of Blood 46-47
      • Tireless Worker 48
      • Four Chambers 48
      • Four Valves 48-49
      • Diastole and Systole 50-51
      • Two Coronary Arteries 52-53
      • Congestive Heart Failure 54-55

   2. *Conduit System*, the Blood Vessels 56-63

      • Arteries 56-58
      • Capillaries 59
      • Veins 60-63

   3. *Transport Medium*, the Blood 64-67

Beneficial Blood Clotting, Embolic Obstruction of Blood Flow, and Harmful Blood Clotting 68-71

Atherosclerosis -- the Most Frequent Abnormality that Affects Our Arteries 72-83

   1. General Considerations 72-76

   2. The Two Main Complications 77-83

      • *Blockage* of Flow Channel 78-81
      • *Aneurysm* Formation 82-83

Introduction

Few assets are more valuable than good health, a precious gift we seldom fully appreciate until we lose it.

In the pages ahead you will learn how to keep your heart and blood vessels healthy. This book will be a joyful adventure in learning how to live a long, healthy, and happy life free of the ravages of arterial disease (*hardened inner walls and flow-surface clots*) that cause **heart attacks, sudden cardiac death, congestive heart failure, strokes, high blood pressure, kidney failure, limb loss, and ruptured aneurysms.**

We will explain how the most common fatal disease processes in the Western world -- *hardening of the arteries and clot formation* -- cause many arteries to *block off* and lesser numbers to *blow out*. We will present a highly effective step-by-step plan to prevent this from happening to you. But if preventive measures haven't been adequate, we will show you how damaged arteries can be repaired or replaced by surgery.

When the blood levels of some types of cholesterol and other fats are high, these chemicals (called lipids) diffuse into the inner portion of the arterial wall. This causes plaques (thickenings) and ulcers to develop which cause clots to form that block the flow channel. Calcific deposits occur around some plaques and make them hard. The popular name for this condition is *hardening of the arteries;* the medical terms for it are *atherosclerosis* and *arteriosclerosis*.

Plaques thicken the arterial wall, narrow the flow channel, and may make the flow surface rough and ulcerated. Plaques may be hard or soft. Many soft ones remain small.

Oily, gruel-like, fatty material may form in the center of the soft plaques. This lipid core is often covered over by a dangerously thin cap of fibrous tissue which is prone to rupture. If this happens, the greasy material contained in the core drains into the flow channel where it can cause the **blood to clot** (a process whereby fluid blood becomes like soft "Jell-O"). This change blocks the artery. Should the cap of a **soft plaque** in a coronary artery of your heart **rupture**, you could die. **This is the most common cause of heart attacks.** Though less frequent, heart attacks are also caused by clots which form on the diseased flow surfaces of hard plaques.

In fewer people, atherosclerosis affects the arteries differently, especially the aorta (the biggest artery). Instead of *blocking* the flow channel, atherosclerosis so weakens the aortic wall that the blood pressure stretches it and forms thin-walled enlargements called *aneurysms* which may rupture (blow out) and cause fatal hemorrhage.

Nearly 45% of all deaths in the industrialized world are caused by blocked arteries and aneurysms due to atherosclerosis (Fig. 1). This staggering total is greater than the sum of those who die from all types of *cancer*, *accidents*, and *infections* combined. Heart disease, in fact, is the most common cause of death in both women and men.

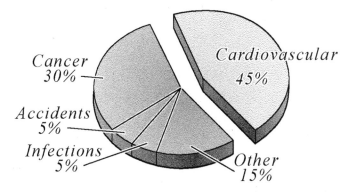

Figure 1 - Causes of death in the United States.

But before you become pessimistic about the ominous threat of *atherosclerosis* and *clot formation* which causes **95%** of the deaths due to heart attacks and strokes in the Western world, there is *good news to tell*. *Proper application of the preventive measures described in this book* (Sections III and IV) *could prevent up to 90% of these premature deaths.* (Please *see* pages 192-194.) And there are many other benefits. A heart-healthy (fit) lifestyle will prevent nearly all cases of lung cancer and emphysema, and most cases of obesity, type 2 diabetes (pp. 279, 280), blindness, kidney failure, and lower extremity amputation.

If preventive measures are applied too late or prove inadequate, there is still hope since most arteries damaged by hardened (diseased) inner walls and clots or by aneurysm formation can be repaired or replaced surgically. Even so, patients undergoing surgery must take the best possible care of themselves for the rest of their lives to obtain optimal results. This is so because surgery is only a mechanical solution to a structural problem. Surgery doesn't correct the underlying biochemical abnormalities that cause the inner arterial wall to harden and clots to form on its flow surface.

Our **primary goal** in this book is to help you keep your arteries (the lifelines within us, Fig. 2, p. 7) free of blockages and blowouts so you will remain healthy (or become so if you aren't now), live a long life, and avoid much medical expense.

To assist you in doing this, we will first consider three subjects that will help you to better understand your body. These subjects are the *cell,* the *life cycle,* and the organization of the body into *11 major organ systems*. **We consider this broad base of knowledge essential for you to develop a heart-and spirit-healthy life style that will enable you to take charge of your health.**

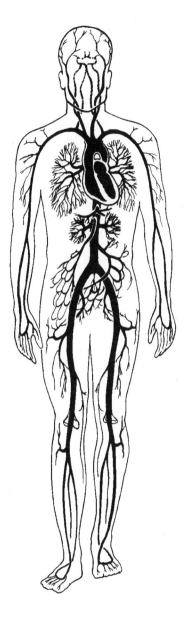

Figure 2 - *"The Lifelines Within Us" --*
Our Arteries

The Cell

Cells are the smallest organized units of life. They are the building blocks from which all tissues and organs are formed. Cells float in a clear, water-like liquid called interstitial fluid. Each cell is a unique world unto itself. About 100 trillion (100,000,000,000,000) cells form our adult physical structure of which 100 billion are brain cells and 100 billion are fat cells.

Oxygen fuels the chemical reactions required for cells to perform their complex functions. Nerve cells discharge electric impulses. Muscle cells contract. Stomach cells secrete digestive juices. Each type of cell has its own special function (Fig. 3, p. 9).

The outer border of the cell is formed by a membrane composed largely of phospholipids, a special type of fat containing phosphorous. This fatty composition makes the membrane insoluble in water and enables it to contain the watery contents of the cell. The membrane's other essential job is to selectively regulate what goes in and out of the cell. Oxygen, water, nutrients, and other chemicals go in, while carbon dioxide and other waste products come out.

The inside of the cell is formed of a soft, semi-fluid "Jell-O"-like material called *cytoplasm*. Located throughout the cytoplasm are many structures including those called *ribosomes* that make proteins, and others called *mitochondria* which produce the energy required by the cell. A round body in the central part of the cell, called the *nucleus*, is formed of even more specialized "Jell-O"-like material which is also surrounded by a fatty membrane. Within the nucleus there are about 50,000 specialized collections of the chemical regulators of life, the **DNA** (**d**eoxyribo**n**ucleic **a**cid) molecules, called *genes*.

Genes are DNA molecules that start, direct, and stop life. They are grouped into specific aggregates called *chromosomes*, which divide when a cell reproduces. The new cells have the same number of chromosomes as their parent cells. Each chromosome is formed of an extremely fine, uniquely folded chromatin strand, which, when straightened out, is about two inches long. If the chromatin strands forming all the body's chromosomes were placed end to end, they would reach to the sun and back about 750 times!

Some Different Cell Types

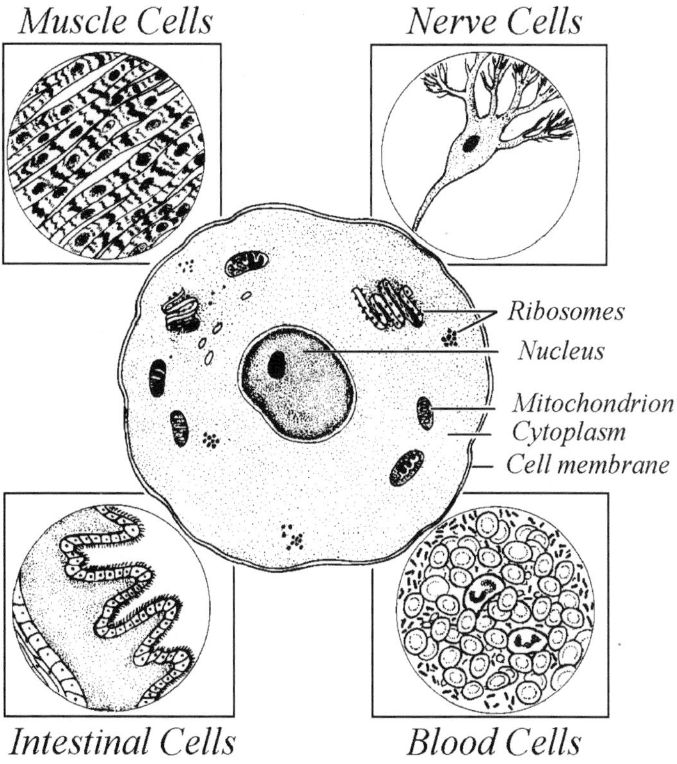

Muscle Cells   Nerve Cells

Ribosomes
Nucleus
Mitochondrion
Cytoplasm
Cell membrane

Intestinal Cells   Blood Cells

Figure 3 - Schematic representation of a "typical" cell and of various cell types. Only four of the many different structures inside the "typical" cell are shown.

The nucleus of every cell of our body has 46 chromosomes, except for the ovum of the female and the sperm of the male, which have 23. The DNA of each gene sends a chemical signal of ribonucleic acid (*RNA*) into the cytoplasm to direct the ribosomes to make one specific protein.

Through these RNA signals (messengers), the DNA of the genes directs the manufacture of all the body's proteins, whether for function, growth, or replacement of worn-out parts. Proteins form the enzymes which direct the production of complex chemicals involving fats and carbohydrates.

The DNA in the chromosomes is also responsible for the perpetuation of life itself by giving the ovum and the sperm the ability to unite and reproduce the species.

Each cell that forms must be nourished by the blood which the heart pumps through the circulatory system.

We will discuss the arteries, capillaries, and veins that make up this system in detail later (pages 56-63). For now, we will simply say that the systemic *arteries* carry red blood away from the left side of the heart and deliver it to the tiny blood vessels called *capillaries* which wind in and out of the minute spaces between the body's innumerable cells.

Oxygen, water, nutrients, and other chemicals in the blood pass through the thin walls of the capillaries into the clear fluid in which the cells float. From there, these life-sustaining materials diffuse into the cells. Waste products, including carbon dioxide, diffuse from the cells in a reverse sequence into the blood, now blue, at the far end of the capillaries (Fig. 4, p. 11). From here, the blood flows on into the systemic *veins* which return it to the right side of the heart.

Capillaries

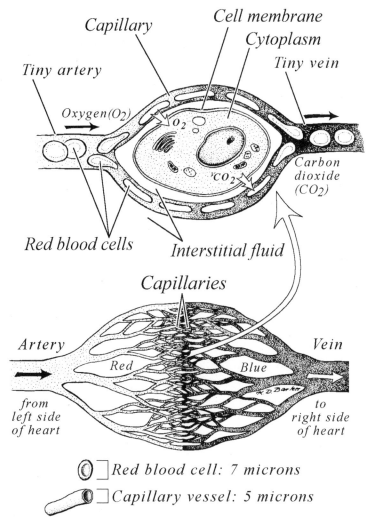

Capillary · Cell membrane · Cytoplasm · Tiny vein · Tiny artery · Oxygen(O_2) · O_2 · Carbon dioxide (CO_2) · CO_2 · Red blood cells · Interstitial fluid

Capillaries

Artery · Red · Blue · Vein · from left side of heart · to right side of heart

Red blood cell: 7 microns
Capillary vessel: 5 microns

Figure 4 - Capillary blood nourishes the cells and removes waste products from them. Red blood cells are bigger than the capillary vessels and must elongate to pass through single file. Absence of a nucleus (p. 64) facilitates this shape change. The red blood becomes blue as it goes through the capillaries and gives oxygen to the cells.

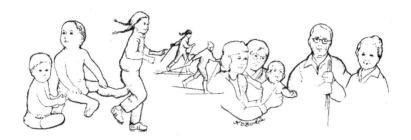

The Life Cycle

The human body is a wondrous result of human and divine creation. It arises from the union of the two generative cells -- one male, the *sperm,* and one female, the *ovum* -- to form one fertilized cell called the *zygote,* whose inception signals the beginning of a new human life. This fertilized cell attaches to the protective tissue of the inner wall of the uterus known as the "endometrium." There the miracle of creation continues for nine months through an incredible sequence of cell division and cell specialization (Fig. 5) into 11 major systems. Then, the human infant is born, totally dependent on others for every care and necessity of life.

After birth, the infant's body continues to develop and grow as its cells multiply throughout infancy, childhood, and adolescence until the adult stage is reached at about 20 years. At that time the body weighs 20 to 25 times more than at birth and is composed of approximately 100,000,000,000,000 (100 trillion) cells. In terms of our planet's population, we have about 20,000 *times* more cells in our body than there are people in the entire world. Yes, hard to believe -- but true.

Even harder, in the early weeks after conception, new brain cells are formed at the rate of about 250,000/minute.

The Life Cycle

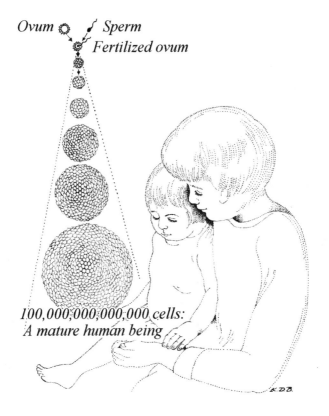

Figure 5 - Our life cycle is a mystery beyond compare -- two cells unite to become one which divides to become two, and those two become four, and those four become eight, and those eight become sixteen, etc., etc., etc., to become a developing entity recognizable as human by four weeks with all the major organ systems taking form. The cells develop in different ways. Some become heart cells, others brain cells, still others bone cells, etc. The growth process continues in a miraculously precise and orderly manner, leading to the birth nine months after conception of a completely helpless, infinitely complex human infant.

Our cells float in a sea of a type of salt water. Water accounts for about 60% of our body's weight. A 200-pound man has about 120 pounds of water (14.4 gallons) in his body. About 10 pounds (1.2 gallons) are in his blood. About 30 pounds (3.6 gallons) are in the fluid in which his cells float. About 80 pounds (9.6 gallons) are in his cells.

Without water to drink, we would live only a few days. We're not as dependent on water as fish, but we come close.

Even more amazing than the development of our physical body is the development of our spiritual self that determines what kind of person we become. The proper development of the spiritual and emotional side of our lives requires that we receive *love* and *protection* in our early formative years.

Our brain is more complex and has greater ability than any computer. If the brain's emotional circuits are established in the first two years for hate and rage instead of for love and peace, they will be very hard to change later.

Neglected and abused children often develop selfish and possessive circuitry in their brains that causes them to become unhappy adults, frequently with little sense of either compassion or justice. **These deficiencies are the root cause of many of the world's current problems.** In fact, the future of our country and the world depends on the love we have for our children and one another. Love, not money, will determine what happens to our human society.

Our children's physical development is determined by *heredity*, *diet*, *exercise*, and the *habits* they learn. As parents we can't change the first factor, but we can change the others because we are responsible for every care in their early formative years. As our children grow and develop, our role becomes more and more one of providing direction and guidance to their lives by the *example* we set for them.

After we become adults, our physical condition depends largely on how we take care of ourselves. We can allow our bodies to become overweight and weak, or we can live our lives in a heart-healthy (fit) manner to enable most of us to live enjoyably into advanced years at low medical expense.

Atherosclerosis, a deadly degenerative disease that affects the inner wall of our arteries, is the leading killer in the U.S. and other industrialized nations. This disease causes the inner arterial wall to degenerate at a markedly accelerated rate. It also causes clots to form on the diseased flow surfaces which can block the arterial channels to the heart, brain, and other vital organs. In addition, atherosclerosis can also cause the arterial walls to weaken, distend, and rupture.

But there is hope! Most people can prevent this hardening process from developing or, if it is already present, from advancing, by choosing to live a heart-and spirit-healthy life.

The prime purpose of this book is to assist you, your children, and grandchildren in this vital selection process.

If we make the proper choices for a heart-healthy (fit) life (pp. 191-195), most of us will reach advanced years in a vital manner, enjoying each day of our earthly journey as we do so.

But we need to recognize the obvious, as Dr. H. Leon Greene states on page 310, that "even a perfect lifestyle will not prevent the inevitable . . . we will all ultimately die." Accordingly, we should also prepare in our own time and way for this transition to eternity, remembering that *physical death is the vital connecting link to all that lies beyond.*

The 11 Major Body Systems

We are more than a mere mass of cells. We are so much more. We are human and possess profound physical, mental, and spiritual dimensions. Our physical components are a marvel of technical efficiency with control mechanisms far more exacting than those of any machine.

As humans, we begin at conception, grow, are born, continue to grow, work, reproduce, mature, age, and eventually die. In this incredible journey we move, sleep, breathe, eat, drink, see, feel, hear, smell, taste, talk, sing, dance, maintain our temperature, digest our food, eliminate wastes, replace parts that wear out, heal injuries, and much more.

And our mental and spiritual dimensions are even more mysterious and grand. They enable us to learn, read, write, develop wisdom, *love*, make decisions, create, feel deeply, compose music, write poetry, record history, appreciate, forgive, see a divine purpose in our lives, feel a closeness to God, and ever so much more.

Differing from all other living species on earth, we humans find happiness by doing for others out of love. Only man is so endowed. Each day of our lives is an opportunity to help our fellow man, and, in doing so, to bring joy into our own lives.

We are a marvel of creation, set apart from all else on earth. And how can all this be . . . **from just two cells that become one**? We are as mysterious as the vast universe in which we live.

In the formative days of our life before birth, the dividing cells of our developing structure differentiated into the innumerable cell types which then went on to form the 11 major systems of our bodies. We will now consider the broad outlines of these miracles of creation in the sequence listed below. Then we will devote special attention to the cardiovascular system in order to appreciate how it serves every one of the 100 trillion cells that comprise our mature physical being. **The 11 major body systems are:**

1. Musculoskeletal System

2. Nervous System

3. Cardiovascular System

4. Hematopoietic (Blood Cell Forming) System

5. Lymphatic/Immune System

6. Respiratory System

7. Digestive System

8. Urinary System

9. Endocrine System

10. Reproductive System

11. Integumentary (Skin) System

We believe that understanding the structure and function of the human body will help all of us live a heart-healthy (fit) life. The most practical way to gain this essential knowledge is to consider the essence of these 11 systems of the body (Figs. 6-16).

1. The Musculoskeletal System

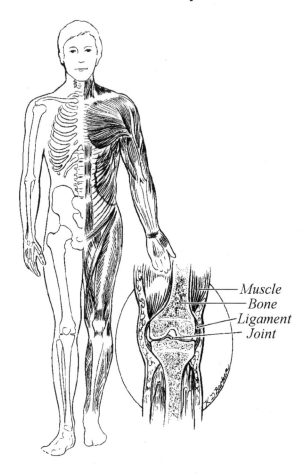

Muscle
Bone
Ligament
Joint

Figure 6 - The musculoskeletal system provides us with form and, in concert with the nervous system, the ability to move. Bones interconnect with other bones through movable connections known as "joints." Muscles arise from a bone on one side of a joint and attach to the bone forming the other side of the joint. When these muscles are stimulated to contract (shorten) by the nervous system, our bones and joints move and this motion enables us to walk, run, jump, and dance.

2. The Nervous System

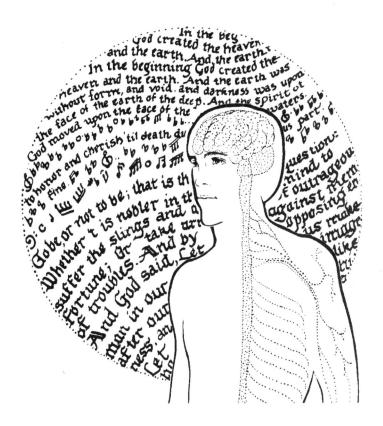

Figure 7 - The nervous system, composed of the brain, spinal cord, and nerves, provides us with the ability to feel, move, balance, see, hear, smell, think, remember, and much more. But of all our wonderful human capacities, our emotional and intellectual capabilities are the most mysterious, such as our capacity to say "I love you," feel compassion, know right from wrong, admit error, ask for forgiveness, write books, identify problems, provide solutions, invent machines, play music, have a sense of destiny, pray, and seek a close relationship with our God.

3. The Cardiovascular System
an Overview

The cardiovascular system has three main parts:
1. A **heart** that pumps 40 million times a year.
2. A vast network of **vessels** that, if placed end-to-end, would form a tube approximately 60,000 miles long.
3. The **blood** that fills the system (about 6 quarts).

There are two sets of three types of vessels -- arteries, capillaries, and veins -- that interconnect through the right and left sides of the heart to form a continuous figure-eight circulatory pathway. One set of vessels, called the *pulmonary circuit*, carries blue blood to the lungs and red blood from the lungs. The other set of vessels, called the *systemic circuit*, carries red blood to the cells and blue blood from the cells.

Arteries start out big at the heart, give off branches, and become progressively smaller (Fig. 8, p. 21). *Capillaries* are tiny; they nourish the cells. *Veins* start out small, join together, and get progressively bigger as they get closer to the heart.

Arteries carry blood away from the heart to the capillaries; veins carry blood from the capillaries back to the heart.

The majesty of the human body is symbolized by the vastness of the blood vessel system through which the right side of the heart pumps the blue blood to the lungs and the left side of the heart pumps red blood to the cells of the body. The red blood supplies all the cells with the oxygen, water, nutrients, and other chemicals they need to survive and function while the blue blood removes the carbon dioxide and other waste products from the cells.

This amazing system is presented in detail on pages 44-67.

Arteries of the Body

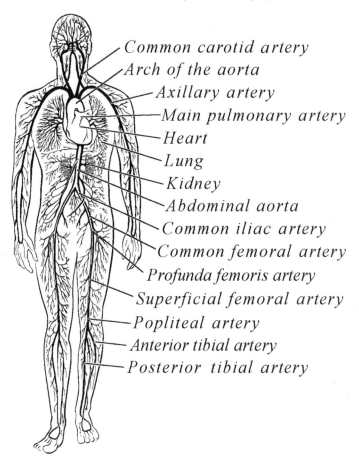

Common carotid artery
Arch of the aorta
Axillary artery
Main pulmonary artery
Heart
Lung
Kidney
Abdominal aorta
Common iliac artery
Common femoral artery
Profunda femoris artery
Superficial femoral artery
Popliteal artery
Anterior tibial artery
Posterior tibial artery

Figure 8 - The arterial system. The right side of the heart receives the oxygen-depleted blue blood returning through the systemic veins (not shown) from the body, and pumps it through the pulmonary arteries into the capillaries of the lungs where it takes up oxygen, gives off carbon dioxide, and again becomes red. The left side of the heart receives this red blood returning through the pulmonary veins from the lungs and pumps it through the systemic arteries into the capillaries of the body where it gives oxygen to and removes carbon dioxide from the cells and again becomes blue.

4. The Hematopoietic
(Blood Cell Forming) System

The hematopoietic system produces the cells and cell fragments found in blood. These include the *red* blood cells that carry oxygen; the *white* blood cells (granulocytes*, lymphocytes, and monocytes) that protect us from infections and cancer; and the *platelets* (tiny pinched-off portions of a big bone marrow cell called a *megakaryocyte*) that stop bleeding and promote healing. These cells and the platelets are formed in the honeycomb-like tissue called *bone marrow* that fills the inside of our bones (Fig. 9, p. 23).

The life span of a red blood cell is about four months; a neutrophilic granulocyte (the common type of granulocyte), several hours to a few days; different lymphocytes, months to years; monocytes, 1 to 2 days; and platelets, 10 days. About 2.5 million red blood cells, 0.5 million white blood cells, and 1.5 million platelets wear out each second and are replaced by an equal number of new ones. And there are many other such balances in our incredible bodies.

Consider for a moment that even if Ford, DaimlerChrysler, and General Motors were combined, they could not make one car per second. This is so, even though making a Cadillac car is less complex than making a single red blood cell.

Blood is composed of about 40% cells and 60% fluid. Most of the cells are red, while a small percentage are white. The fluid, called *plasma,* contains special chemicals -- sodium, potassium, calcium, magnesium, oxygen, carbon dioxide, proteins, fats, carbohydrates, cholesterol, vitamins, enzymes, hormones, and many more. The beating heart pumps the blood through the vessels so that it can nourish all the cells of the body with what they need to survive and function.

* **cyte = cell (from the Greek)**

The Hematopoietic
(Blood Cell Forming) System

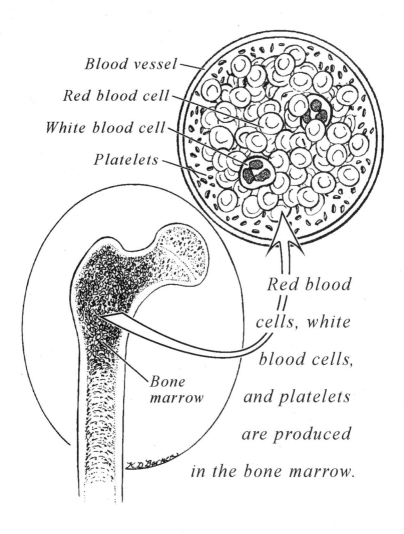

Blood vessel

Red blood cell

White blood cell

Platelets

Red blood cells, white blood cells, and platelets are produced in the bone marrow.

Bone marrow

Figure 9 - The red blood cells, white blood cells (granulocytes, lymphocytes, and monocytes), and platelets are formed inside our bones in the honeycomb-like tissue called bone marrow.

5. The Lymphatic/Immune System

The lymphatic system consists of thin-walled *lymph channels*, about 1000 interspersed collections of lymphatic tissue *(lymph nodes)*, clear fluid called *lymph* (filtered out from the blood) that flows slowly through this system, and *lymphocytes* (cells that circulate in the blood and lymph). The lymph returns to the blood through a big lymph channel which joins a large vein at the base of the neck on the left side. **The lymph system has three important functions:** first, to *protect* us from infections and cancers; second, to continuously *refresh* the fluid that the tissue cells float in; and third, to *transport* digested fat from the bowel to the blood.

The immune system consists of the *lymphatic system*, *spleen*, and *thymus* (Fig. 10, p. 25). These three components protect the body from bacteria, viruses, fungi, and cancer cells. The spleen is about the size of an open hand and is located in the upper left portion of the abdomen. The thymus is located in the upper front part of the chest directly behind the breast bone. It is very large in infancy, but shrinks with age, becoming largely replaced by fat in the adult.

Some lymphocytes make special proteins called *antibodies* that attack bacteria, viruses, fungi, and cancer cells. These proteins circulate in the blood where they lock onto the surface of these invaders and kill them. Most importantly, these lymphocytes continue to make these specific protein weapons for long periods, often for many years. For example, the vaccine for smallpox is composed of a weak virus that causes only a mild reaction. But this mild reaction gives the vaccinated person immunity for several years from being infected with the strong virus that causes the severe disease.

The Lymphatic/Immune System

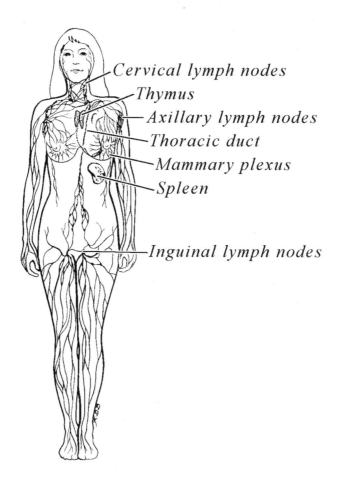

Figure 10 - The lymphatic/immune system is a vital defense mechanism for our body. Loss of a portion of it -- as occurs in advanced AIDS -- is usually fatal within a year or two from infections with bacteria, viruses, fungi, and often from the development of cancer, as well (p. 66).

6. The Respiratory System

The respiratory system (Fig. 11, p. 27) is composed of *three parts*: an upper, a middle, and a lower airway. This system has two main functions: first, to provide oxygen to and remove carbon dioxide from the blood; and second, in concert with the nervous system, to enable us to speak.

The *upper airway* consists of the nose and pharynx. The *middle airway* consists of the larynx (voice box) and the trachea (windpipe) and its two divisions (right and left main bronchi), and, in turn, their major subdivisions. The *lower airways* (lungs) consists of increasingly smaller air passages which branch into approximately 600,000,000 tiny, one-cell thick air sacs (alveoli) that have a combined surface area of about 2,000 square feet (71% the size of a tennis court). The alveoli are covered on their outer surfaces by tiny blood vessels (*capillaries*) that are only one cell thick. Oxygen passes in and carbon dioxide passes out through these walls.

The oxygen content of the air in the alveoli is higher than the oxygen content of the blue blood in the capillaries, while the carbon dioxide content of this blood is higher than that of the air in these tiny sacs. When we breathe in, oxygen diffuses from the air sacs into the blue blood and turns it red, while carbon dioxide diffuses from the blood into the air sacs. The exchange of these gases in the lungs enables the circulating blood to *carry oxygen to* and *remove carbon dioxide from* all the cells of the body.

The incredible balance of nature is exquisitely shown in the way plants and animals use air. Animals use oxygen and make carbon dioxide in the oxidative chemistry of living, while plants use carbon dioxide and make oxygen in the photosynthetic chemistry that enables them, and us, to live.

The Respiratory System

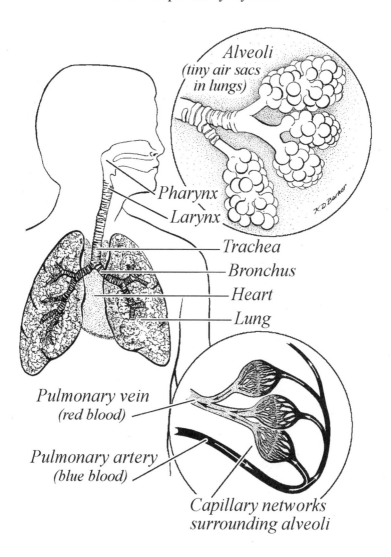

Figure 11 - This system is constructed to provide a massive surface for interface of the oxygen-depleted blue blood (returning from the body) with the atmosphere. In this reaction, the blood surrounding the tiny air sacs takes up oxygen from the air to become red and gives off carbon dioxide into the air sacs.

7. The Digestive System

The digestive system (Fig. 12) is composed of a tube about 30 feet long (small intestines about 20 feet) that meanders from mouth to anus through the core of our bodies, and two glands (one large - the pancreas, - and the other huge - the liver). The tube functions as a "conveyor belt" that is loaded at the mouth with food and water. The digestive process begins by chewing and swallowing. The ingested food and water are moved along by the massaging, undulating, forward motion of the "belt" known as *peristalsis*. This peristaltic activity "stirs" the food "mix" and assures its contact with the powerful digestive enzymes secreted by the glands of the mouth, stomach, duodenum, pancreas, and small intestines (bowel). As this happens, the food is digested into ever-smaller chemical units.

The dense covering of the inner surface of the small intestines by villi (tiny projections) provides a surface area equal to that of five tennis courts. This huge surface enables the pancreatic and other enzymes to function efficiently, converting carbohydrates into simple sugars, fats into fatty acids, and proteins into amino acids. These basic subunits are absorbed by the intestinal wall. Simple sugars and amino acids are carried by the blood to the liver. Fatty acids and chylomicrons (particles of emulsified fat) are carried by the lymphatics to the blood and then to the liver. The pancreas also secretes hormones (insulin and glucagon - p. 35) directly into the blood to regulate the blood glucose.

The liver (weighing about four pounds) is the body's giant chemical factory. It receives raw materials from the small intestines and makes them into innumerable vital compounds to supply all the cells of the body. The liver also excretes *bile*, a greenish fluid, into the duodenum through the bile duct. The gall bladder, an out pouching of the bile duct, stores bile and, after we eat, empties it into the duodenum to assist digestion. The peristaltic action of the small intestines (jejunum and ileum) moves the indigestible portions of our food (along with excess water, bile, matter excreted by the intestinal glands, cells shed from the surface of the intestines, and friendly bacteria) into the large bowel (colon and rectum), and finally through the anus to the outside of the body as a "bowel movement."

The Digestive System

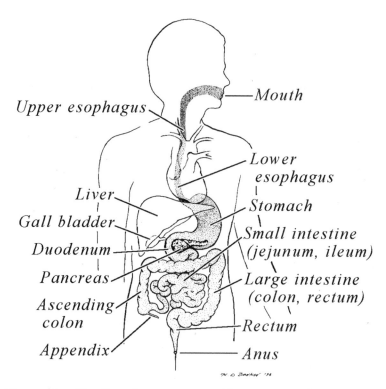

Figure 12 - The digestive system provides a vast surface (greatly increased by the villi) upon which our food is broken down into its basic components that are absorbed into the blood and lymph and carried to the liver for further chemical processing.

8. The Urinary System
(With Comments About the Artificial Kidney and Kidney Transplantation)

The urinary system (Fig. 13) is composed of two kidneys, each connected by a drainage tube *(ureter)* to the bladder where a single drainage tube *(urethra)* empties to the outside.

Each kidney has about one million filtration units (nephrons) containing an approximate aggregate of 45 miles of fine tubules that are a marvel of chemical efficiency. These structures remove waste products, excess water, and extra minerals from the blood; selectively concentrate them; and then excrete what's left as a yellow fluid called *urine*.

If the kidneys stop functioning, death usually occurs within a few days due to toxic elevations of potassium in the blood that cause the heart to stop. Should the kidneys fail, their function can be taken over by a machine that "washes," *i.e.*, "dialyzes" the blood or by an exchange method that puts fluid into the abdomen and removes it a few hours later. These methods enable large numbers of patients with no function of their own kidneys to live for many more years.

If a suitable donor kidney for transplantation becomes available and the patient's condition is satisfactory, a transplant may be possible. Unfortunately, this logical solution to a very large medical problem is inadequate because there are many more patients in permanent kidney failure who require chronic treatment with the artificial kidney for continued life than there are donor kidneys that are suitable for transplantation. There are about **10,000 kidney transplants** done each year in the U.S. The need is far greater. These patients are anemic, too, because they don't secrete enough of the red blood cell stimulating hormone, *erythropoietin* (p. 102).

The Urinary System

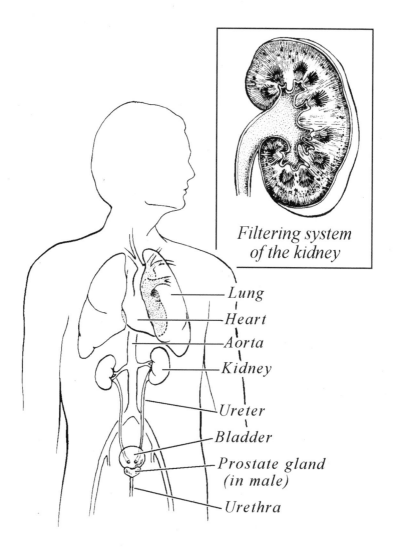

Lung
Heart
Aorta
Kidney
Ureter
Bladder
Prostate gland (in male)
Urethra

Filtering system of the kidney

Figure 13 - To keep the water content and chemistry of the blood in balance, the kidneys filter about one quart of blood each minute.

In the U.S. today, nearly 200,000 patients with chronic kidney failure are able to live reasonably normal lives because of the artificial kidney. These patients, who would otherwise die within days, are attached to an artificial kidney three times a week for periods of three to four hours. During that time about 2/3 of a pint of their blood is run through the machine per minute, removing waste products, excess water, and minerals from it. This "washing" of the blood is called *hemodialysis*.

The connections to the machine are established by placing two large needles into a vein in the forearm, one to bring the patient's blood to the machine which "washes" it and the other to return the "washed blood" back to the patient. The bigger this vein and the stronger its wall, the better it can function for hemodialysis.

The best way to develop such a vein is to make a direct surgical opening between an adjacent artery and vein near the wrist. The blood in the high pressure artery rushes through this opening into the low pressure vein and causes it to become enlarged and thick-walled all the way up the forearm.

These changes in the vein are essential if it is to be used successfully for hemodialysis treatments three times a week over a long period of time. During the first year alone, the vein must be punctured by big needles at least **312 times!**

But if a suitable direct connection can't be made between an adjacent artery and vein, it may be possible to place an artificial blood vessel graft between an artery in one part of the forearm and a vein in another part. In this instance, the needles are placed into the artificial graft.

When possible, the direct connection of an artery to a vein is preferred for hemodialysis access because such a vein will usually function for a much longer time before closing off than will an artificial graft. Some veins may function for 10 to 20 or more years.

Some patients can't use hemodialysis because they have no suitable veins that can be punctured to establish connections with the kidney machine. For these patients, a procedure called *continuous ambulatory peritoneal dialysis* can be used instead. An advantage of this technique is that the patients can be up and about while the dialysis exchange is taking place in their abdomens.

In this method, 2 to 3 quarts of dialysis fluid are run through a special connector into the peritoneal cavity (the space in the abdomen that contains the stomach, bowels, and liver) where it is left for several hours and then drained out. More fluid is added. The cycle is repeated 3 to 4 times a day. At bedtime, the fluid is replaced, left in overnight, and drained out in the morning. This repetitive cycle is continued day in and day out.

During the time the fluid is in the peritoneal cavity, waste products, excess water, and extra minerals diffuse into the fluid and are removed when it is drained out. Though less efficient than hemodialysis, peritoneal dialysis is preferred by patients who wish to self-administer their dialysis treatment at home. The peritoneal method is easier than hemodialysis for them to learn and carry out.

The dramatic evolution of the science of treating kidney failure has led to the medical specialty of *nephrology* and to the surgical specialties of *hemodialysis* and *kidney transplant surgery*. Today, few people die of kidney failure in the developed countries of the world because of dialysis.

9. The Endocrine System

The endocrine system (Fig. 14, p. 35) is made up of a series of glands (pituitary, thyroid, parathyroid, adrenals, islet cells of the pancreas, ovaries in females, and testicles in males) that make special chemicals called *hormones* which are secreted directly into the bloodstream where they circulate to distant organs and influence their function in vital ways.

For example, the *pituitary gland* (located inside the skull) is called the "master" gland of the body, because it secretes hormones that control the function of the other endocrine glands. It also secretes a hormone that controls growth and another that enables the kidneys to reabsorb needed water from the filtration tubules. Without this latter hormone, we would die from loss of water within a few hours.

The *thyroid gland* (located in the neck) secretes a hormone called *thyroxine* which regulates the body's metabolic rate. This hormone determines how fast our "motor" runs.

The *parathyroid glands* (located behind the thyroid) secrete a hormone called *parathyroid hormone* that controls the calcium content of our bodies, which in turn influences the beat of the heart, the contraction of muscles, and the structure of bones.

The *adrenal glands* (located atop the kidneys in the back of the upper abdomen) secrete several hormones; one of these, called *adrenaline,* enables us, in times of stress or danger, to get that instant acceleration we need to react beyond our usual capacity. Other adrenal hormones, such as *cortisone* and *aldosterone,* control much of the vital chemistry of life relating to stress, minerals, sugar, and water.

The pancreas (located in the back of the upper mid-abdomen) contains about two million tiny clusters (called "islets") of endocrine cells (alpha and beta types) that secrete hormones. The alpha cells secrete *glucagon* which causes the glycogen (p. 274) to release glucose when more energy is needed. The beta cells secrete *insulin* (p. 274) which enables our cells to use glucose for energy and, when there's an excess, to store it as glycogen in liver and muscle cells (p. 274). But, if the glycogen sites are full, this excess glucose is converted into saturated fat. In diabetics, insulin is absent or ineffective (pp. 279, 280).

The *ovaries* (located in the pelvis) secrete "estrogens" and "progesterone" and the *testicles* (located in the scrotum) secrete "testosterone." These hormones make the genders different.

The Endocrine System

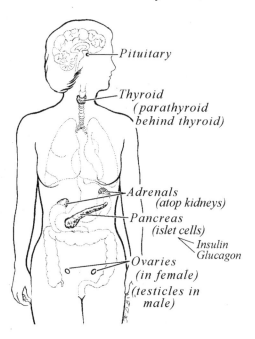

Figure 14 - The endocrine system controls the chemistry of our bodies. Without its hormones, we would die in minutes.

10. The Reproductive System

The reproductive system provides the two cell sources
(ovaries in the female for the ovum, and testicles in the male
for the sperm) upon which the continuation of the human race
depends (Fig. 15, p. 37).

The remainder of the reproductive anatomy in both the male
and female is pertinent to the union of these two cells to form
a fertilized ovum that develops within the uterus into that
most remarkable of all earthly mysteries, the *human infant*.

The reproductive system has the dual purpose of continuing
the human race and, in my personal belief, of being involved
in the expression of mutual love in the married state between
husband and wife.

There is no responsibility more awesome than that of
parenthood. My wonderful wife has been an inspiration to
each of our eight children and, now, as grandmother to our 23
grandchildren. By loving care and direction, parents can
guide their children to become responsible, loving, happy
adults. In this light, Robert Browning reminds us that a world
devoid of love would soon become a desolate tomb.

The home and family are the foundation of our human
society and the basis of what is most precious in our lives. We
need to appreciate and nurture this truth each day by showing
our love, starting at home.

In time, our children will take over from us and run the world
of tomorrow while we move on to eternity. Preparing them
for these resposibilities is up to us. This continuum of life
speaks to a divine order.

The Reproductive System

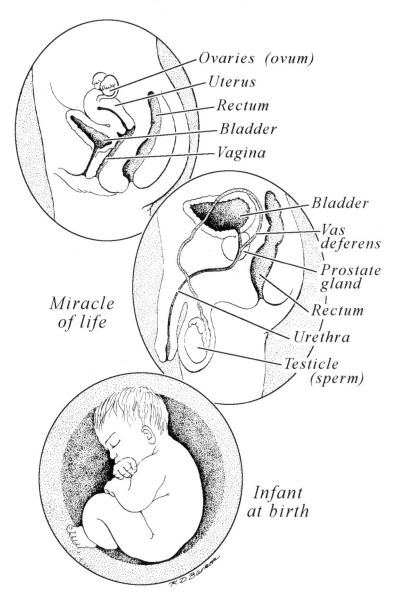

Ovaries (ovum)
Uterus
Rectum
Bladder
Vagina

Bladder
Vas deferens
Prostate gland
Rectum
Urethra
Testicle (sperm)

Miracle of life

Infant at birth

Figure 15 - The reproductive system is responsible for the continuation of human life on this planet (Figs. 6-16).

11. The Integumentary (Skin) System

The integumentary system comprises the outer covering of our bodies, and so to speak, we live within it (Fig. 16, p. 39). Although few people think of the skin as an organ, it is actually the largest (and in many ways the most unusual) organ of the body. The average adult man has about 20 square feet of skin, while the average woman has somewhat less.

The skin has **three vital functions:** first, to *keep* the underlying tissues from drying out (serving like the peel of an orange or the skin of an apple); second, to *prevent* bacteria, viruses, and fungi from invading our bodies; and third, to *maintain* our body temperature within a precise zone. To facilitate this latter function, the skin has approximately 2 million sweat glands. The skin is so important that if these functions are impaired or lost over a substantial portion of the body, as from a major burn, the patient may die despite the best medical care.

Heat is produced by the chemical reactions ongoing in each of our 100 trillion cells. Our body temperature is kept nearly constant at 98.6 degrees Fahrenheit (37 degrees Centigrade) so that the enzymes and chemcial reactions of our cells can function in an optimal manner. Maintenance of this critical balance is achieved by regulation of the amount of heat that is lost through the skin. This is accomplished by precise control of two complex functions: the volume of blood flowing through the deeper layer of the skin and the amount of sweat evaporating from the surface of the skin.

The greater the volume of blood flow through the skin, the greater will be the loss of heat from its surface, provided that the temperature outside the body is less than the temperature inside. If it is greater, we must depend on sweating for cooling.

When the weather is hot and the generation of heat within the body is high, as during exercise, the sweat glands of the skin become active. As this sweat evaporates, the heat of vaporization is taken largely from the surface of the skin, cooling it (and the body) in the process.

The Integumentary (Skin) System

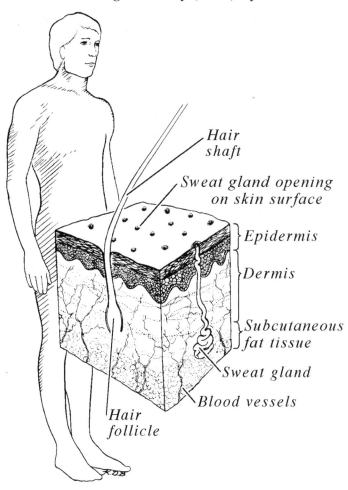

Figure 16 - The integumentary system protects us from the outside world and keeps our body temperature at 98.6°F.

The "Boundary Organ" Concept

Let us now consider how the circulation of blood through our vessels, the *lifelines* within us, sustains the 100 trillion cells of our bodies by providing them vital contact with the outer environment through the lungs, intestines, liver, kidneys, and skin (Fig. 17, p. 41). In this broad context, these organs make up an exchange zone where oxygen, water, nutrients, and other chemicals are brought into the body, and carbon dioxide, other waste products, and heat are removed from it.

The needs of every cell of our bodies must be taken care of by these boundary organs. Blood is the vehicle that enables this vital metabolic commerce to occur.

What and how much we eat is critically important to this exchange. There are three basic food types: carbohydrates, fats, and proteins (*see* p. 137 and the glossary). In brief, carbohydrates (4 calories/gram) are used for energy; fats (9 calories/gram) are a vital component of every cell's walls and are also used for energy; and proteins (4 calories/gram) form the muscles (engines), enzymes (regulators), tissues (structures), and cell components (machinery) of our bodies.

The heart pumps the blood through the lungs, intestinal tract, and liver where it receives oxygen, water, nutrients, and other chemicals from the outside world. The blood then carries these supplies to the body's cells where they are utilized in the chemical reactions of life that generate energy and heat, repair damaged parts, and synthesize new compounds. The waste products of these reactions pass into the blood that delivers them to the lungs, liver, kidneys, and skin which discharges them to the outside as components of breath, bile, feces, urine, sweat, and heat.

The "Boundary Organ" Concept

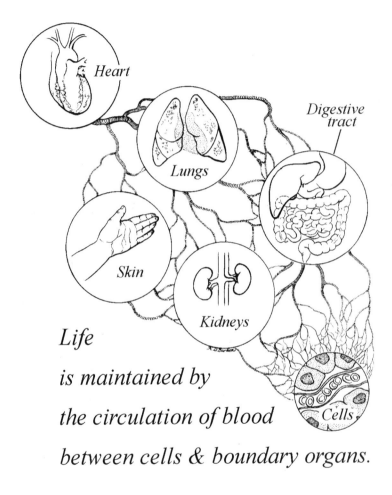

Heart

Lungs

Digestive tract

Skin

Kidneys

Cells

Life

is maintained by

the circulation of blood

between cells & boundary organs.

Figure 17 - The boundary organ concept asserts that for the cells of the body to survive, they must all have contact with the outside world. Without water, we would die in several days; without food, in several weeks. The circulation connects our cells to the boundary organs (lungs, intestines liver, kidneys, and skin) where the metabolic exchange occurs. In this manner, the cells obtain what they need and discharge what they don't need.

The Lungs

In the lungs, respiratory gases are exchanged with the atmosphere. When we breathe in, fresh air fills the tiny air sacs of the lungs and enables oxygen to diffuse into the blue blood flowing through the capillaries that surround the alveoli. In these capillaries, oxygen combines with hemoglobin (the iron-containing protein in the red blood cells) to form *oxyhemoglobin,* a bright red compound, which turns the blue blood red. As this is happening, the blood releases carbon dioxide which diffuses into the air sacs. When we breathe out, this "stale" air with its load of carbon dioxide and decreased amount of oxygen is expelled from our lungs into the outside air.

Oxygen is needed to fuel the chemical reactions in each cell. These reactions produce carbon dioxide which would become harmful if high concentrations were to develop. This does not occur because the venous blood continuously transports carbon dioxide from the tissues to the lungs where the excess is exhaled to the outside world (pp. 26, 27).

We breathe faster and more deeply during strenuous exercise to supply our muscles with the added oxygen they need and to remove the extra carbon dioxide they produce. Precise control mechanisms regulate these adjustments.

Our crucial dependence on a continuous supply of oxygen to our cells is shown by what would happen if our hearts were to suddenly stop beating (p. 275). We would lose consciousness in about 10 seconds. In fact, we would be "out" before we hit the floor because our brains would go blank before our muscles would lose their tone and cause us to collapse. And **by four minutes**, many of our brain cells would be damaged beyond repair from lack of oxygen.

The Small Intestines and the Liver

The small intestines are like a grocery store where the cells of the body place their orders for food and water. In a real sense, they are at our mercy because their selection is limited to what we provide them by the diet we eat and drink. *They have to take what we give them!* What we force our arteries to "consume" can harden their inner walls and cause clots to form that block the flow of blood to such vital organs as the heart and brain. *Hardening of the arteries and clot formation kill more people in the Western world than any other cause.*

In the intestines, food is chemically broken down, combined with water, absorbed by the blood (carbohydrates and proteins) and lymphatics (fats), and *carried to the liver for chemical processing.* Then the blood, now loaded with chemicals, flows from the liver to the heart and lungs, and is pumped on to the tissues to supply the needs of all the body's cells for oxygen, water, nutrients, and other chemicals.

The Kidneys

Waste products are produced constantly in our cells and are carried by the blood to the kidneys, where most are excreted in the urine along with excess water and minerals to keep our body's chemistry in proper balance.

The Skin

The skin functions as a huge radiating and vaporizing surface to release the excess heat generated by the chemical reactions in the body's cells into the outer environment at a rate that will keep our body temperature nearly constant at 98.6° F (37° C). This precise temperature regulation is essential for the optimal function of the innumerable enzymes that regulate the vast number of chemical reactions ongoing in our cells.

The Cardiovascular System
Detailed Examination

Three Main Parts

The three main parts of the cardiovascular system are:
1. **Power source**
2. **Conduit system**
3. **Transport medium**

The *power source,* the **heart,** is an almost inexhaustible muscle that contracts (beats/pumps) over 100,000 times each day. No other muscle can do so much work. The *conduit system* is a huge network of **vessels** that if placed end to end would wrap twice around the earth at the equator and extend for an additional 10,000 miles (Fig. 18). The *transport medium,* the **blood,** through the contracting power of the heart and vast scope of the distribution system, reaches all of the body's 100 trillion cells and supplies their needs.

Vascular System

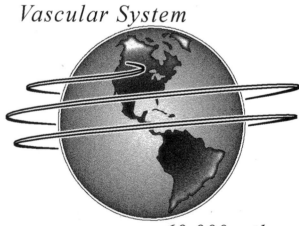

60,000 miles

Figure 18 - The blood vessels of one person if placed end to end would encircle the earth at the equator nearly 2.5 times.

1. Power Source -- The Heart

The heart is a muscle pump (with valves) that beats in a
rhythmic manner to propel blood through an incredible
system of vessels to supply the body's 100 trillion cells. Our
life depends on the continuous flow of blood from heart to
cells and back again in a never ending cycle (Fig. 19, below).

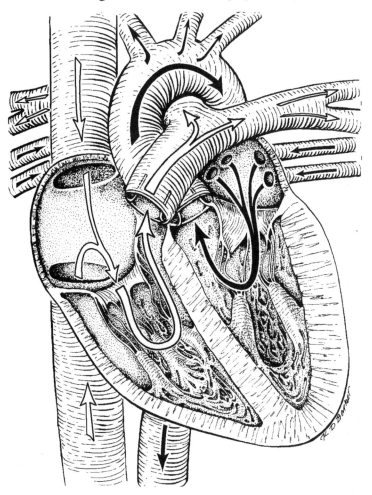

Figure 19 - The Human Heart.

Circulatory Cycle
and
Color Changes of Blood

The circulatory pathway of the blood is composed of a figure-eight circuit with one loop (the systemic) for the body and one loop (the pulmonary) for the lungs. Each loop has an arterial and a venous component connected by a capillary bed. The blood is blue in the systemic veins and pulmonary arteries and red in the pulmonary veins and systemic arteries (Fig. 20, p. 47). The blue color indicates a lower oxygen content and the red color a higher oxygen content.

The right side of the heart receives the blue blood returning through the systemic veins from the body and pumps it on through the pulmonary arteries into the capillaries of the lungs where it combines with oxygen and turns bright red. This red blood flows on through the pulmonary veins into the left side of the heart which pumps it forward through the systemic arteries into the tiny capillaries that supply the 100 trillion cells of the body with oxygen. The color of the blood turns "blue" as this happens. This blue blood flows back through the systemic veins into the right side of the heart, completing the circulatory cycle. **If this cycle stops, we die.**

The blue blood turns red in the capillaries of the lungs when oxygen combines with the dark-blue-colored, reduced hemoglobin (pp. 284,285) in the red blood cells to form the bright-red-colored *oxyhemoglobin*. Then, as the arterial blood gives up part of its oxygen to the cells, the blood becomes blue again. The more oxygen the red cells give up to the tissues, the darker (more blackish) these cells and the blood become. In this process, *hemoglobin*, a complex protein, is the "vehicle" that loads up with oxygen in the lungs and delivers it to the cells.

Color Changes of Blood

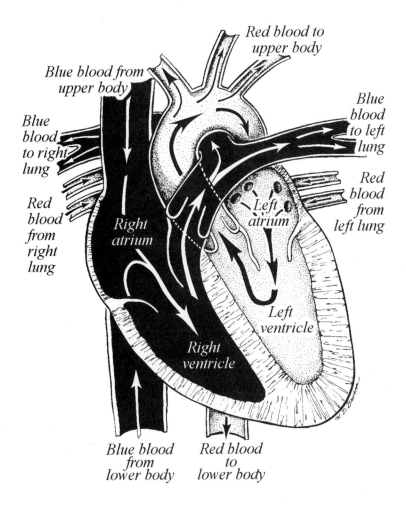

Blue blood from upper body

Red blood to upper body

Blue blood to right lung

Blue blood to left lung

Red blood from right lung

Red blood from left lung

Right atrium

Left atrium

Left ventricle

Right ventricle

Blue blood from lower body

Red blood to lower body

Figure 20 - Arrows indicate the circulatory pathways of the blue blood (shown as black) returning from the body to be pumped by the right side of the heart to the lungs and the circulatory pathways of the red blood (shown as stippled) returning from the lungs to be pumped by the left side of the heart to the 100 trillion cells that comprise our physical bodies.

Tireless Worker

The heart is the power source for life -- a blood pump that can never rest. The heart beats about 80 times/minute (faster during exercise and slower during sleep), 4,800 times/hour, 115,000 times/day, 40 million times/year, and one billion times in 25 years.

During maximal exercise the heart pumps up to four to six times what it does at rest, with most of the blood going to the working muscles. Even calculated on resting output alone, the adult heart pumps about 1-1/2 gallons of blood/minute, 90 gallons/hour, 2,200 gallons/day, 800,000 gallons/year, and 56 million gallons in 70 years (equal to what the mighty Amazon empties into the Atlantic in one second).

Four Chambers

On the right side, the heart has a receiving chamber (right atrium) to receive the blue blood returning from the tissues (depleted of oxygen and laden with carbon dioxide) and a pumping chamber (right ventricle) to pump it to the lungs. On the left side, the heart has a receiving chamber (left atrium) to receive the red blood returning from the lungs (replenished with oxygen and depleted of carbon dioxide) and a pumping chamber (left ventricle) to pump it back to the tissues to supply the cells.

Four Valves

The heart must have well-functioning valves to work efficiently: two inlet valves to open when the ventricles are ready to fill and two outlet valves to open when the ventricles are ready to eject (Fig. 21). Thus, the heart has four valves, an inlet valve and an outlet valve for both the right and left ventricles. The inlet valves are the *tricuspid* on the right and the *mitral* on the left. The outlet valves are the *pulmonary* on the right and the *aortic* on the left. If these valves don't open or close properly, the heart muscle must do extra work to pump the volume of blood that is required to adequately nourish all the body's cells. Diseased valves are like bad gears; they cause trouble.

Valves of the Heart

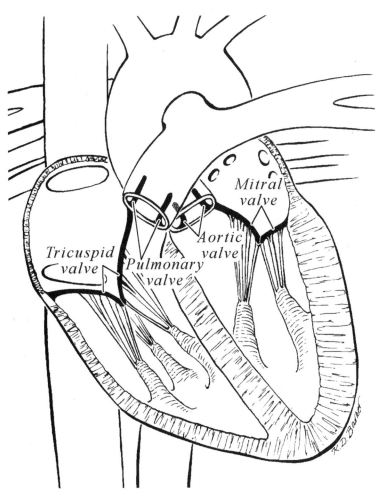

Figure 21 - Heart has four valves. When normal, they work like magic.

Diastole and Systole

Diastole is the blood-filling phase of the heart beat (Fig. 22, below). The heart must fill before it can empty. In diastole the inlet valves (tricuspid and mitral) open as the outlet valves (pulmonary and aortic) close, allowing the blue blood from the body to flow into the right ventricle and the red blood from the lungs to flow into the left ventricle.

Heart in Diastole

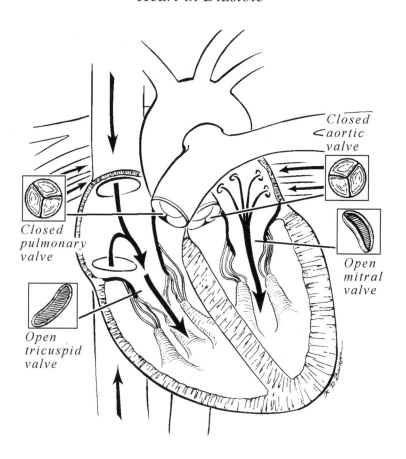

Closed
< aortic
valve

Closed
pulmonary
valve

Open
mitral
valve

Open
tricuspid
valve

Figure 22 - Filling of ventricles in diastole.

Systole is the contracting or pumping phase of the heart beat (Fig. 23, below). As the ventricles begin to contract, their inlet valves (tricuspid and mitral) close and shortly thereafter their outlet valves (pulmonary and aortic) open as the pressures in the respective ventricles rise above those in the pulmonary artery and aorta. The continuing contraction of the right ventricle pumps the blue blood to the lungs while that of the left ventricle pumps the red blood to the body.

Heart in Systole

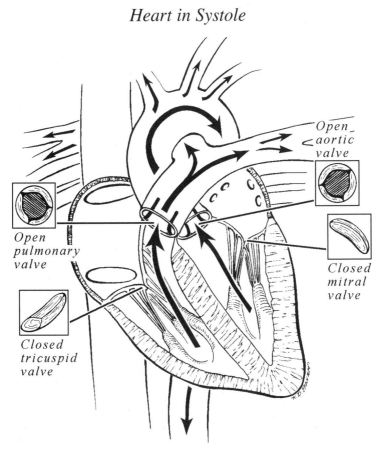

Open aortic valve

Open pulmonary valve

Closed mitral valve

Closed tricuspid valve

Figure 23 - Emptying of ventricles in systole.

Two Coronary Arteries
- The Heart's Fuel Lines -

For the heart muscle to do its work, the muscle must be nourished by an adequate supply of well-oxygenated (red) blood. This "high-octane fuel" reaches the muscle cells through two arteries, called the *right* and *left* coronaries (Fig. 24, p. 53).

The left coronary is about 1/4 inch in diameter where it originates from the aorta, while the right is usually a little smaller. These two arteries, the first branches of the aorta, receive about 5% of the blood that the heart puts out at rest.

If the heart's entire blood supply were to be suddenly cut off, the beat would become weak and ineffective within a minute or two and would soon stop completely. For the heart to work, it must receive oxygen and nutrients. This means it needs an adequate supply of red blood.

The volume of red blood that flows through our coronary arteries depends on our level of activity and varies from about 1/2 pint per minute at rest to 2 to 3 pints per minute at maximum exercise.

The heart, which weighs only about 2/3 of a pound (roughly 0.4% of the body's weight), consumes about 10% of the oxygen used by the entire body, even though, when contracted, it's only about the size of your fist.

Both of the *coronaries* have two main branches, which in turn have branches, and these branches branch, etc. In developed, industrialized countries, blockage of the coronary arteries from atherosclerosis and clot formation kills nearly as many people as all other causes of death combined.

Coronary Arteries of the Heart

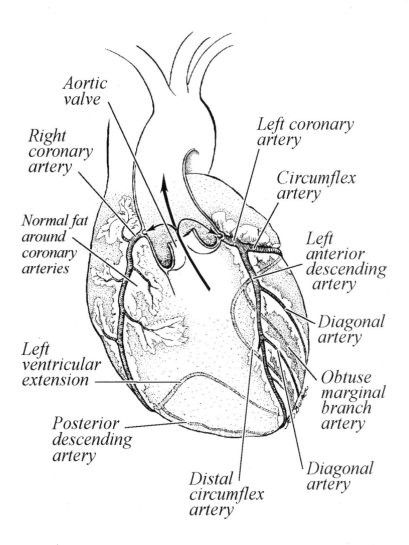

Figure 24 - Heart is nourished by two coronary arteries, a right and a left.

Congestive Heart Failure

The failing heart can't pump enough blood to enable the body's cells to function properly. The most frequent causes of this condition are decreased blood supply to the heart muscle due to coronary artery disease (atherosclerosis) and clot formation, reduced numbers of adequately functioning muscle cells as a result of heart attacks (due to coronary artery disease), impaired valve structure (causing either obstruction, leakage, or both), high blood pressure (hypertension), viral infections of the muscle cells of the heart, and excessive intake of alcohol .

No matter the cause, heart failure makes the patient weak because the tissues don't receive enough oxygen and nutrients to do their work. If the left ventricle fails, the blood backs up into the lungs and causes them to fill with water. This forces the exhausted patient to fight for each breath. If the right ventricle also fails, the blood backs up into the brain, liver, intestines, abdomen, kidneys, and legs, causing them to swell. Congestive heart failure is an agonizing way to die -- breathless, weak, confused, nauseated, unable to eat, and compelled to sit up and gasp for air (Fig. 25, p. 55).

Fortunately, congestive heart failure can often be improved by medicines which cause the kidneys to excrete more salt and water, by diets that restrict salt intake, by drugs which increase the strength of the heart beat, and by agents that expand the small arteries and decrease the blood pressure. If heart failure is due to abnormal valve function or to lack of coronary blood supply, surgery to correct these problems may be very beneficial. But for patients with worn-out hearts, transplantation is their best chance for recovery. The problem is that there are many more patients dying of heart failure than there are donor hearts available for them. This is why there is a pressing need for a permanent artificial heart.

Person in Congestive Heart Failure

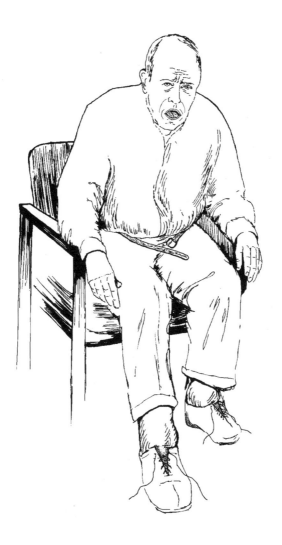

Figure 25 - This individual has failure of both the left and right sides of the heart. He is weak, gasping for breath, and unable to lie down because his heart can't pump enough blood. The tiny air sacs of his lungs are full of water, and his brain, liver, intestines, abdomen. kidneys, and legs are also waterlogged and swollen.

2. Conduit System -- The Vessels

We have three types of blood vessels -- arteries, capillaries, and veins. The structure of these vessels in the pulmonary and systemic circuits is similar, though the walls of the systemic arteries are thicker (blood pressure is 5-6 times higher in systemic arteries). The systemic arteries carry the red blood pumped by the left side of the heart to the capillaries which deliver oxygen, water, nutrients, and other chemicals to the cells. The blood, now blue, receives waste products from the cells. The systemic veins return this blue blood to the right side of the heart which pumps it through the pulmonary arteries into the alveolar capillaries where it takes up oxygen, loses carbon dioxide, and turns red. This blood flows on through the pulmonary veins into the left heart.

Systemic Arteries

Arteries are relatively thick-walled tubes made up of three different layers of tissue (Fig. 26) that surround a channel (lumen) through which the blood flows to the capillaries. From a functional standpoint, arteries connect the heart to all the cells of the body. They are indeed the *lifelines* within us.

The *innermost layer* is the thinnest and is called the *intima*. It's lined with delicate cells called *endothelium* which are in direct contact with the blood flowing through the lumen.

The *middle layer* is the thickest and is called the *media*. It is made up of alternating circular sequences of elastic fibers, smooth muscle cells, and collagen fibers.

The *outermost layer*, called the *adventitia*, is composed of loose fibrous tissue containing small blood vessels called the *vasa vasorum* (vessels of the vessels) that penetrate the outer portion of the media and nourish its cells.

The cells of the intima and the inner portion of the media to a depth of about 1/50 of an inch are nourished by diffusion of oxygen, water, nutrients, and other chemicals from the red blood flowing through the lumen. Beyond that depth the wall is nourished by the red blood flowing through the vasa vasorum. In veins, these tiny vessels extend much closer to the flow surface than they do in arteries.

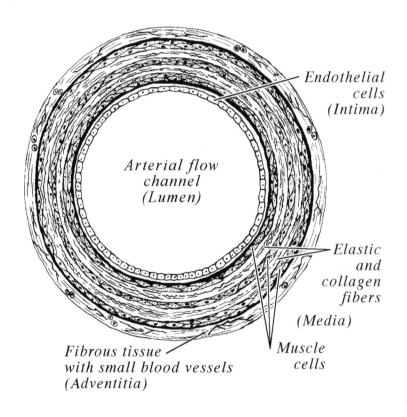

Figure 26 - Cross Section of a Systemic Artery.

In systole when the heart contracts (Fig. 23, p. 51), the right ventricle pumps blue blood to the lungs and the left ventricle pumps red blood to the body. This increases the pressure which causes the large arteries to dilate and elongate.

The dilation and elongation of these big vessels in systole enables them to hold more blood. Between beats while the heart fills (Fig. 22, p. 50), the elastic recoil of the distended arteries propels blood to the lungs and the rest of the body.

The combination of hardening of the arteries (p. 72) and clot formation is by far the most common cause of death in the industrialized world. If an artery becomes blocked as a consequence of this disease, the tissues that it nourished will likely die from lack of oxygen and nutrients.

No one knows why atherosclerosis develops so often in the bigger systemic arteries but rarely does so in some smaller ones, such as the *internal mammary arteries* inside the front of the chest, and almost never develops in the tiny arteries.

The aorta, the biggest artery, is, in a sense, like the trunk of a tall tree. The trunk rises up from the roots (the heart) and has many branches. These branches branch and their branches, branch in turn, becoming progressively smaller as they do so. The main trunk gets smaller as this branching occurs. At the level of the navel, the trunk divides into two large branches of equal size called the common iliac arteries, each of which divides again on either side of the pelvis to supply blood to the lower half of the body.

The arteries branch until they are so tiny that they can only be seen with a high-power microscope. Then, they connect with the vast sea of still tinier vessels called *capillaries* (Fig. 27, p. 59) that nourish the 100 trillion cells of the body.

Systemic Capillaries

The capillaries -- incredible in number and microscopic in size (Their wall is but one endothelial cell thick, and their channel is less than one-tenth the width of the finest human hair.) -- receive the red blood from the arteries and form seemingly endless networks of tiny channels that surround the trillions of cells which make up our bodies (Fig. 27, below). The combined surface area of all the systemic capillaries is about 3,000 square feet, an area slightly larger than that of a tennis court. Each one of the billions of capillaries in our bodies nourishes hundreds of cells. Oxygen, water, nutrients, and other chemicals in the blood pass through the capillary walls into the clear liquid the cells float in and diffuse from there into the cells to supply their needs.

The waste products which arise from the chemical reactions of life that go on in each cell diffuse out into the fluid around the cells. From there, these products pass through the capillary walls into the blood of this vast network of lacy microvessels which merges into the tiny veins that are the beginning of the systemic venous system which returns the blood, now blue, back to the right side of the heart.

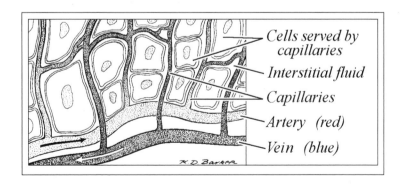

Cells served by capillaries
Interstitial fluid
Capillaries
Artery (red)
Vein (blue)

Figure 27 - The systemic capillaries nourish the cells and remove their waste products.

Systemic Veins

Like arteries, veins are lined by endothelium and are made up of three layers of tissue, but the walls of the veins are much thinner, more supple, and less elastic than those of the arteries (Fig. 28, below). The tiny feeding vessels in the venous wall extend to within 1/1000 of an inch of the flow surface.

The pressure is so low in veins that they don't need thick, muscular walls. This low pressure may be why the systemic veins (and pulmonary arteries and veins) don't develop atherosclerosis. Arteries don't have valves, but arm and leg veins have many valves which prevent the blood from flowing backward when we sit, stand, breathe out, cough, or strain.

The capillaries merge to form tiny veins that progressively join to form fewer but larger veins until there are but two, the *inferior vena cava*, which drains all the blue blood from the lower body into the bottom of the right atrium of the heart, and the *superior vena cava*, which drains all the blue blood from the upper body into the top of the right atrium (Fig. 29, p. 61). From there the right ventricle pumps the blue blood to the lungs, where it receives oxygen and turns red.

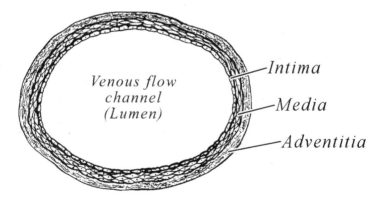

Figure 28 - Cross Section of a Systemic Vein.

Veins of the Body

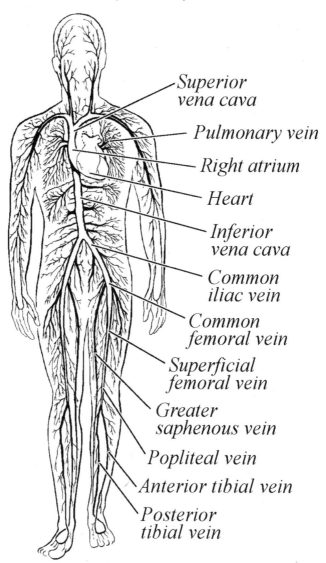

Superior
vena cava

Pulmonary vein

Right atrium

Heart

Inferior
vena cava

Common
iliac vein

Common
femoral vein

Superficial
femoral vein

Greater
saphenous vein

Popliteal vein

Anterior tibial vein

Posterior
tibial vein

Figure 29 - The systemic veins return the blue blood (low oxygen content) from the tissues of the body to the right side of the heart and the pulmonary veins return the red blood (high oxygen content) from the lungs to the left side of the heart.

The forces that cause the blue blood to flow back from the tissues to the right side of the heart are:

1. The force from behind, the small residual energy remaining from the heartbeat.

2. The force of gravity in the erect position on the blood returning from the head and neck.

3. The suction force created by increasing the dimensions of the chest during inspiration.

4. The pumping force developed in the veins by the intermittent contraction of the surrounding muscles, especially those of the calf, during walking, running, dancing, or simply moving the ankles up and down when standing, sitting, or reclining (Fig. 30, p. 63).

If the venous valves work well, contraction of the calf muscles squeezes the thin-walled veins running between them. This propels the blood in these veins toward the heart as the valves below the compression site close, and those above it open. Relaxation of the calf muscles expands the compressed veins. This closes the valves above, opens those below, and literally sucks the blood up from the lower tissues (Fig. 30, p. 63).

The calf muscles function like an auxiliary pump for the venous blood. This helps to move the blood back to the heart and decreases the blood's tendency to clot. This is why physicians advise patients to move their feet and ankles while in bed after surgery.

The Venous Pump

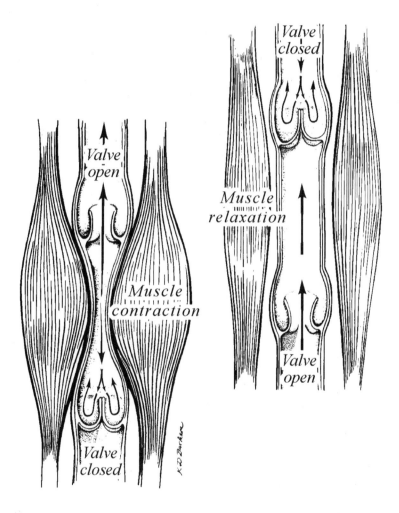

Figure 30 - Contraction of calf muscles during walking pumps the venous (blue) blood back to heart against gravity. If the venous valves leak, this process is inefficient.

3. Transport Medium -- The Blood

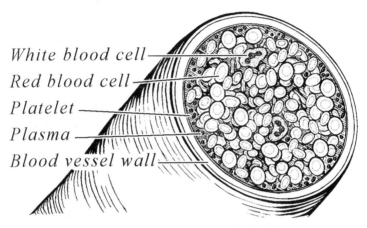

White blood cell

Red blood cell

Platelet

Plasma

Blood vessel wall

Figure 31 - Composition of Blood.

The blood is a majestic substance made up of about 40% free-floating cells and 60% fluid. Just imagine the difficulties of having to design a liquid that could carry the vast array of chemicals and huge number of cells required to nourish, regulate, and defend the trillions of cells that make up our physical bodies. Further, the blood must also be able to fill and flow easily through the 60,000 miles of blood vessels in each of our bodies. This distance is nearly 2.5 times the circumference of the earth at the equator, and is 75 times the length of the Alaska Pipeline. *And yet the average person has only about six quarts of blood with which to fill this system.* Incredible -- but true!

The blood has huge numbers of red cells that carry oxygen to the tissues; lesser numbers of white cells (granulocytes, lymphocytes, and monocytes) that combat infection; and large numbers of cell particles, called platelets, that stop bleeding and promote healing (Fig. 31, above). The red blood cells, the only cells in the body that don't have a nucleus, lose theirs a short time before they are released from the bone marrow.

The number of cells in the blood staggers the imagination. Conventionally, the "blood count" is expressed as the number of cells present in one cubic millimeter (mm^3) of blood. To put this into better perspective, consider what is contained in one teaspoon of blood.

One teaspoon of blood (5,000 mm^3) contains approximately:

25,000,000,000	red blood cells
20,000,000	granulocytes (white cells)
10,000,000	lymphocytes (white cells)
2,000,000	monocytes (white cells)
1,250,000,000	platelets

If the bone marrow were to make too many red blood cells, the blood would become like sludge and cause our hearts to fail. If the marrow formed too few, we would die because our blood would be unable to carry enough oxygen.

The blood cells are suspended in the fluid component of the blood which is called *plasma*. This remarkable fluid transports these cells with their chemicals plus all the other chemicals that are essential for our survival.

When an invasion of bacteria occurs into the tissues (acute infection), the tissues release chemicals that cause the bone marrow to release a flood of white cells *(granulocytes)* into the blood. These defenders, attracted by chemicals in the tissues, stream into the invasion area, such as a lung with pneumonia or the back of the neck with a boil, and attack the invaders. The white cells attempt to kill the bacteria by engulfing them, while the bacteria try to kill the white cells with toxins they produce. As the battle rages on, the area of combat becomes red, hot, swollen, and tender. Medically, this warfare between the white cells and the invaders is called *inflammation*.

The successful development of medicines to poison bacteria that invade the body started with the discovery of the sulfa drugs in the late 1930s. This development sharply tilted the balance of force against these invaders. Unfortunately, over time many bacteria have developed resistance to antibiotics that would have killed them a few years ago. Because of this, research teams are working intensively to develop new antibiotics to which these resistant bacteria are sensitive.

Lymphocytes protect us from infections and cancer. These cells arise in the thymus, spleen, lymph nodes, and bone marrow. Some lymphocytes defend us by making *antibodies* (special proteins that kill specific invading bacteria, viruses, fungi, and cancer cells), while other lymphocytes defend us by attacking these agents directly.

In the development of *AIDS* (Acquired Immune Deficiency Syndrome), the Human Immunodeficiency Virus *(HIV)* invades the nucleus of the lymphocytes and directs these cells to produce the deadly virus instead of making antibodies to fight the infection. Lymphocytes die, and, at the same time, their production falls. When the lymphocyte count drops to a critical level, the patient develops debilitating, chronic infections, and often cancer, too. Now, largely defenseless, the patient can't fight back and usually dies within a year from the ravages of this disease, despite intense supportive care.

Enormous research effort is being directed to develop both an effective medical treatment and a vaccine against this dreaded disease. The need for a major breakthrough in this research is urgent because the worldwide AIDS epidemic continues to grow, especially in third-world countries. Fortunately, some progress is now being made, providing hope for the future. But high drug costs are a major problem, especially in sub-Saharan Africa.

Monocytes are cells formed in the bone marrow and spleen that are essential for the healing of a wound, prevention of infection, and recovery from injury. They engulf bacteria and matter that needs to be removed in order for healing to occur, and they also release growth factors that continue the healing process initiated by the platelets.

Some monocytes migrate into the vessel wall and others go completely through it to become large tissue cells called *macrophages*. This name means "big eater." These cells devour bacteria, dead tissue, and clots. Like monocytes, macrophages are a rich source of growth factors that continue the tissue reactions until the wound has healed.

Platelets are tiny pinched-off portions of the bulging cytoplasm of a large cell in the bone marrow called a *megakaryocyte*. These cytoplasmic fragments enter the blood stream and are called *platelets,* because they resemble little plates. Most float along in the blood stream near the vessel wall, ever ready, should injury pierce the wall, to stick together (aggregate) and set off a local clotting reaction to close the opening and stop the bleeding. In fact, if we were to stop making platelets, we would soon bleed to death, even from minor injuries. But if we were to make too many, we would clot to death. The production of platelets is regulated by a growth factor, called *thrombopoietin*, which is made in the liver.

In any significant injury, vessels are damaged and some blood is lost into the wound. The platelets in the wound play two vital roles when this happens. First, as mentioned above, they aggregate (stick together), which acts to stop bleeding in the wound; second, they release chemicals called *growth factors* that promote healing. These chemicals attract cells and tiny blood vessels into the wound where they multiply and heal the injury.

Beneficial Blood Clotting, Embolic Obstruction of Flow, and Harmful Blood Clotting

Beneficial Blood Clotting

A clot is a semisolid coagulum of blood. **Beneficial Clotting** is one of the many life-preserving functions of our blood. Without this capability, we would bleed to death from even a small cut. In other words, clotting is a normal, vital, and highly desirable reaction of blood under appropriate circumstances. But *clotting can also occur in the wrong place, at the wrong time, and for the wrong reason -- and can kill us by closing off a vital artery.* This can happen, for example, when the thin tissue cap over the lipid core of a soft plaque ruptures and allows the fatty material to ooze into the blood, where it activates the platelets and causes clotting.

Beneficial clotting in an artery, such as that which occurs when you accidentally cut a finger (Fig. 32, p. 69), is triggered by the activation of platelets by the injured tissues. Platelets are only about 1/5 the width of the red blood cells. Because they are small and light, platelets float along in the outer portion of the bloodstream close to the wall. The blood contains about one platelet for every 20 red cells.

But near the wall, the platelets outnumber the red cells and are ever ready to react to an injury. When the wall is injured, the platelets adhere to the damaged wall and become activated, a process which brings out their inherent maximal stickiness. These activated platelets stick to the injured area and to each other. When other platelets come in contact with these sticky platelets, they also become activated and stick to them. The process continues, forming an aggregate, a ***platelet plug,*** capable of closing a small cut in a little vessel.

But if the cut is too big to be closed by a platelet plug alone, platelets have another property that helps them get the job done (Fig. 32, below). They can cause *fibrinogen,* a protein in the blood, to form strings of an elastic, thread-like, sticky material called *fibrin* which sticks to itself, to the platelets, and to the injured wall, forming a multilayered mesh around the platelet plug that traps red blood cells to form a clot which attaches to the wall and attempts to span the opening. But if the clot is unable to close the opening, surgical care is required to stop the hemorrhage. If such help is not immediately available, the hemorrhage can often be stopped temporarily by applying direct pressure over the bleeding vessel, allowing time for the patient to be transported to a facility (hospital, surgicenter, or office) where this care can be given.

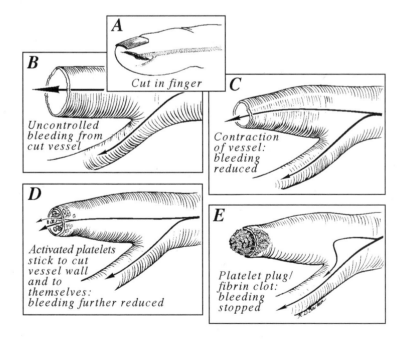

Figure 32 - Platelet plug with fibrin clot stops bleeding.

Embolic Obstruction of Blood Flow

An embolus is a free-floating object that is carried by the blood to where it plugs the channel and blocks the circulation. Emboli may be small and break up quickly to restore blood flow, or they may be larger and persist to cause a major stroke or loss of a limb.

Most arterial emboli are fragments of platelet aggregates, clots, or atherosclerotic debris that break loose and are swept by the blood to where they block the channel (Fig. 33, p. 71). Most venous (pulmonary) emboli are clots that have broken loose from leg veins and are carried by the blood to the lungs where they plug the pulmonary arteries and block the circulation. Some pulmonary emboli are so big that they can cause death in a few minutes.

Harmful Blood Clotting

Though activated platelets can save our lives by stopping bleeding, they can kill us by causing harmful clots and emboli (see above). In this book, we focus our consideration of harmful clotting on that initiated by the diseased inner wall of hardened arteries. In hardened arteries, the diseased inner wall can activate platelets in two ways to cause harmful clots:

1. By contact (as described on p 68) of blood with the fatty liquid that drains from the **lipid core** of a soft plaque when the thin tissue cap over it ruptures (Fig. 34, p. 74).
2. By contact of blood with the mounds of cholesterol, other fatty materials, and calcium which form the irregular, **roughened, ulcerated flow surfaces** of some of the hard plaques in atherosclerotic arteries (Fig. 35, p. 75).

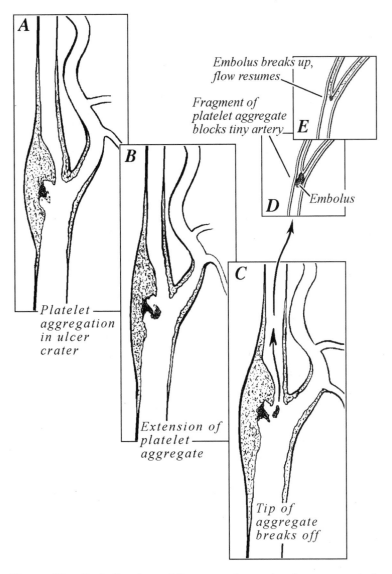

Figure 33 - Embolization of fragment from platelet aggregate in ulcerated carotid plaque to small artery in the brain where it causes loss of function. If the embolus breaks up rapidly, the impairment clears quickly. Such a brief stroke-like episode is called a transient ischemic attack, abbreviated TIA (Fig. 44, p. 98).

Atherosclerosis
-- The Most Frequent Abnormality
That Affects Our Arteries --

1. General Considerations

In general there are *four* conditions that adversely affect our arteries: injury, infection, tumor formation, and hardening of the arteries (atherosclerosis). Injuries are uncommon; infections and tumors are rare. But atherosclerosis is the most frequent cause of disability and death in the affluent Western world.

Atherosclerosis is a metabolic disorder that causes the inner arterial wall to degenerate (pp. 4-6, 15, 73, 77, 78, 272,273).

This diseased inner wall can kill us in one of two ways:
1. More often, it **narrows the arterial channel, and then activates platelets that cause clot formation which completes the closure**, stopping blood flow to vital organs, such as the heart, producing a fatal heart attack.
2. Less often, the process weakens the aortic wall so much it progressively bulges out to form an **aneurysm** that eventually ruptures and causes deadly hemorrhage.

Atherosclerosis is caused by *blood chemistry abnormalities that result from* heredity; smoking; a high-calorie diet of low-fiber carbs, refined sugar, saturated fats, and *trans* fatty acids; a sedentary lifestyle; obesity; diabetes; and undue stress.*
These blood abnormalities include:
1. High levels of one type of cholesterol (LDL - p. 73).
2. Low levels of another type of cholesterol (HDL - p. 73).
3. High levels of triglycerides (blood fats).
4. High levels of blood glucose (diabetes, pp. 196,279,280).
5. High levels of homocysteine* (an amino acid -- p.197).

* **Please see index and glossary for more on atherosclerosis causes.**

High blood pressure, gout, and low thyroid function also predispose us to develop atherosclerosis.

In about 5% of the people who develop atherosclerosis, *genetic* factors cause their abnormal cholesterol chemistry. These people were born with an inability of their livers to remove LDL cholesterol from their blood. **In the other 95% of people with hardened arteries, *lifestyle* factors, are the cause of their disease.**

The terms <u>HDL</u> and <u>LDL</u> stand for high- and low-density lipoprotein, respectively. Union with proteins makes cholesterol, a fat, soluble in the blood and tissue fluids. Because of its greater protein content, HDL cholesterol transports LDL cholesterol and other fats out of the arterial wall to the liver for reprocessing and/or excretion in the bile. But this can't happen if there isn't enough HDL to do the job. For this reason HDL is often called the "good" cholesterol and LDL the "bad" cholesterol even though LDL cholesterol is essential to the life of every cell in the body. But as with all the body's chemicals, safety is a matter of dosage. LDL cholesterol above 130mg/dL is bad (below 100 is ideal).

Excess LDL cholesterol and triglycerides diffuse into the inner arterial wall and cause plaques (areas of scar and necrosis) to form. Calcification of these plaques may occur. If marked calcification develops, the plaque becomes *hard*. If little occurs, the plaque remains *soft*. Many small, soft plaques develop a highly viscous, oily center, called the *lipid (fatty) core*. These soft plaques may rupture and discharge their lipid contents, causing platelets to aggregate and blood to clot. **Coronary occlusion due to rupture of soft plaques (Fig. 34, p. 74) is the most frequent cause of heart attacks**. Ulcerated hard plaques in coronary arteries may also activate platelets, incite clotting, and cause heart attacks (Fig. 35, p. 75).

Rupture of Lipid Core with Clotting

A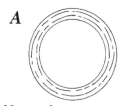

Normal coronary artery.

B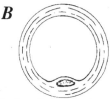

Soft plaque forming.

C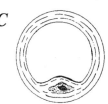

Soft plaque develops fatty liquid in central portion.

D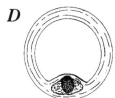

Fatty liquid core expands. Tissue on top becomes thin.

E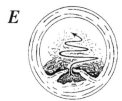

Tissue over top ruptures. Fatty liquid oozes into blood and activates platlets, causing blood to clot.

F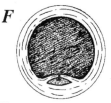

Clotting of blood continues and closes flow channel.

Figure 34 - Development of small, soft plaque with a lipid core in a coronary artery. The core enlarges and ruptures its fibrous cap, allowing the deadly, oily contents to ooze into the blood, causing it to clot. This blocks the flow channel and causes a heart attack, the most common cause of death in the U.S. If a clot-dissolving drug is given within the first hour after the artery closes, it will likely dissolve the clot, restore blood flow, and save the heart muscle.

Ulceration with Clotting

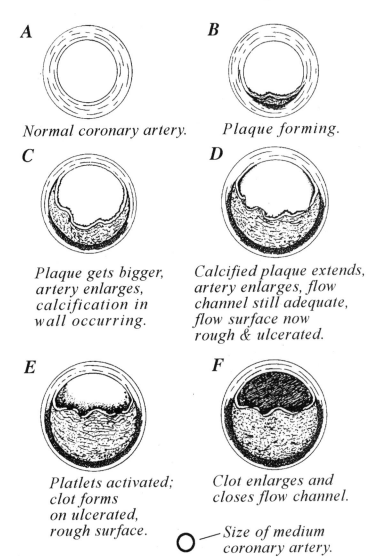

A

Normal coronary artery.

B

Plaque forming.

C

Plaque gets bigger,
artery enlarges,
calcification in
wall occurring.

D

Calcified plaque extends,
artery enlarges, flow
channel still adequate,
flow surface now
rough & ulcerated.

E

Platlets activated;
clot forms
on ulcerated,
rough surface.

F

Clot enlarges and
closes flow channel.

○ —Size of medium
coronary artery.

Figure 35 - Development of hard (calcified) plaque with flow
surface roughening and ulceration in a coronary artery causes
platelets to adhere, activate, and aggregate, inciting clot
formation which blocks the flow channel, causing a heart attack.

Modern life in the U.S. tends to make us stressed, sedentary, and overweight. Advertisements for fast, high-calorie, convenient, tasty foods high in low-fiber carbohydrates, refined sugar, saturated fats, and *trans* fatty acids are always before us. In time, our blood chemistry mirrors whether we smoke, what we eat, how much we exercise, what we weigh, and the degree of stress in our lives.

What we *should* do to preserve our arteries, the *lifelines* within us, is obvious. *We must stop smoking, eat a proper diet, exercise regularly, attain and maintain a healthful weight, and control the reactions to the stress in our lives.* Adopting this simple prescription for heart-healthy (fit) living is the most practical way to stop the epidemic of deaths and disability due to heart disease and many types of cancer, especially of the lung. These diseases are strangling the Western world and, increasingly, the *entire* world.

While we agonize over the high cost of medical care in the U.S., we still subsidize the farming of tobacco, and we fail to educate our children about the benefits of disease prevention. It's time for us as a *nation* to become realistic. We must take action before the exorbitant cost of our medical care escalates to insurmountable heights. We can do this by decreasing the number of people who become patients and need high-tech, expensive medical care. We can make this happen if each of us will commit to the lifestyle choices that will enable us to live as healthily as possible.

There's no doubt -- our arteries are "lifelines." For when they **block off** or **burst**, we suffer severely and may die. Because of this, most of the rest of the book after this section concentrates on the diagnosis, *prevention*, and surgical treatment of these **main complications of atherosclerosis and clot formation**.

2. The Two Main Complications

For emphasis, we repeat and amplify that the two main complications of atherosclerosis and clot formation are *blockage* of the flow channel and *aneurysm* formation. These adverse effects may be summarized as follows:

- **Blockage of the flow channel.** The flow channel of hardened arteries may become narrowed by thickening of the diseased inner wall and closed by clots triggered by platelets, which are either activated by rupture of soft plaques with lipid cores, or by roughness and ulceration of the flow surface of calcified plaques. Such blockage deprives the downstream tissues of vitally needed blood. This lack of blood supply causes heart attacks, strokes, high blood pressure due to decreased flow of red blood to one or both kidneys, blindness, kidney failure, decreased walking capacity, and loss of limbs. These conditions are much more common than aneurysms and occur in highest frequency in diabetic patients.

- **Aneurysm formation.** Here, the wall of the atherosclerotic artery, usually of the aorta in the abdomen about an inch below where the arteries to the kidneys arise, weakens and gives way under the incessant pounding of the arterial pressure to form a balloon-like bulge called an aneurysm. Aneurysms of the aorta continue to get bigger and, usually without prior symptoms, suddenly rupture, causing fatal hemorrhage. For unknown reasons, aneurysms occur more frequently in non-diabetics than in diabetics .

We will now consider how these "block" and "burst" complications develop.

Blockage of the Flow Channel

Atherosclerosis begins when high blood levels of LDL cholesterol, other fats, and homocysteine (p. 197) damage the fragile endothelial cells lining the inside of arteries. The lipids (cholesterol and other fats) then move into the muscle cells in the inner part of the wall and injure them. Some die. Other muscle cells move in from the outer wall, and some of these die, too. Muscle cells around these areas of injury secrete proteinaceous materials to wall them off.

Bone-like, calcified material then forms around some of these deposits, forming what medically is called a *hard atherosclerotic plaque*. Others remain soft and small and some of these develop *viscous lipid cores*. The hard plaques make the wall thick, stiff, and often brittle -- giving rise to the lay term "hardening of the arteries." The thickened inner wall may develop ulcers and clots. Surprisingly, the most frequent cause of harmful clot formation that causes heart attacks is not the hard ulcerated plaque. Instead, it is the small, soft plaque that ruptures, releasing its deadly **lipids** into the blood, where they activate **platelets**. These activated platelets cause clots that block the flow channel (Fig. 34, p. 74). This is the most common cause of heart attacks. Though a less common cause of heart attacks than plaque rupture, harmful clotting also occurs from **platelets** being **activated** by contact with the **ulcerated flow surface** of hard plaques that have lost their protective layer of endothelial cells (Fig. 35, p. 75).

When the main artery to a part of the body is closed off by atherosclerosis and clot formation, the only blood that is able to reach the tissues downstream gets there by going through little branches that arise *above* the blockage and join with small branches that originate *below* it (Fig. 36, p. 79). If this is not enough for survival, the tissues die, such as those of the heart in a heart attack or of the brain in a stroke.

Blockage Due to Atherosclerosis and Clot Formation

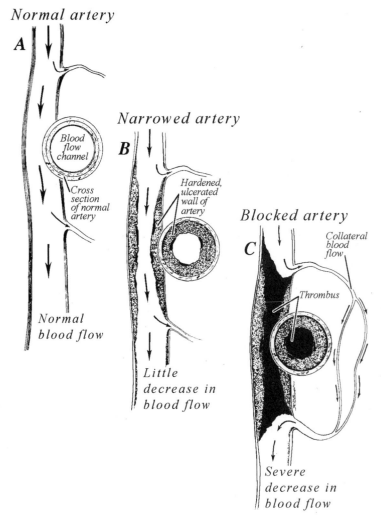

Figure 36 - Progressive Blockage of the Flow Channel. (A) Normal artery with open flow channel. (B) Development of atherosclerosis with thickening of inner wall, narrowing of channel, and ulceration of flow surface. (C) Blockage of channel by clot (thrombus) which has formed on diseased flow surface. Collateral present.

Nature's Attempt to Compensate
for Blockage of the Flow Channel

If the flow channel of an artery becomes blocked *gradually,* the branches that arise immediately above and below the blockage have time to enlarge, grow toward one another, and eventually meet to establish direct connections that provide some blood flow to the tissues downstream.

The vessels that make these connections are called *collateral channels,* and the blood that flows through them is called *collateral circulation* (Fig. 37, p. 81).

Sometimes, if the closure is gradual, these collateral channels may become sufficiently large that when the main artery finally closes, the person never realizes that anything has happened (Fig. 88, p. 242). This is unusual because nature requires a long time to form such large channels.

If complete obstruction occurs quickly, as when a soft, small coronary plaque with a lipid core ruptures and causes the blood to clot, a heart attack usually occurs because there isn't enough collateral circulation to supply the oxygen and nutrients necessary to keep the muscle alive (Fig. 34, p. 74).

Through bypass surgery, a surgeon can rapidly *create* a very large "surgical" collateral vessel by placing a graft from the open artery *above* the obstruction to an open artery *below* it (Fig. 90, p. 244). This creates a big collateral *around* the blockage and supplies needed blood to the "starved" tissues downstream.

The signs and symptoms of a blocked artery depend on: (1) the organ or part of the body that's affected, (2) the severity of the blockage, and (3) the degree of collateral circulation that the body has the time and capacity to develop.

Collateral Circulation
Nature's Strategy for Blockage

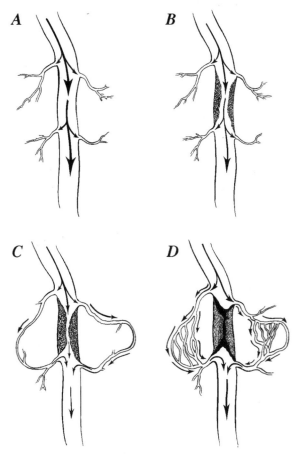

Figure 37 - Development of collateral circulation. (A) Normal artery with small branches, no collateral circulation. (B) Same artery with moderate narrowing due to atherosclerosis, no collateral circulation. (C) Same artery with severe narrowing and ulceration. Collateral developing. (D) Same artery, now completely closed by atherosclerosis and clot formation, with more collateral circulation bypassing the blockage. Occasionally, as shown here, substantial flow develops.

Aneurysm Formation

Even high blood pressure cannot rupture a *normal* artery because its strong elastic wall has plenty of strength to contain the powerful force of the heart beat.

But in some people, *atherosclerosis* weakens the arterial wall so much that the power of the pulse causes the wall to balloon out. This happens most often in the biggest artery, the aorta, more often in the abdomen (about an inch below where the arteries to the kidneys arise) than in the chest, and less often in the arteries of the legs. As the dilated area (aneurysm) gets bigger, the tension on its wall increases. This increasing tension causes aneurysms to enlarge, setting up a vicious circle whereby small aneurysms get big, and big aneurysms get bigger, until they finally burst (Fig. 38, p. 83).

Though the rate of enlargement of an aneurysm of the aorta is usually gradual, with enough time, the wall will **weaken** and **stretch** to the point that the arterial pressure will eventually **rupture** it. When that happens, massive hemorrhage occurs which is quickly fatal unless emergency surgery can be performed to successfully stop the blood loss.

Under the best of circumstances, the death rate for patients undergoing emergency surgery for ruptured abdominal aortic aneurysms is high -- often above 50%. Because of this, surgery by an experienced vascular or endovascular surgeon (p. 202; Fig. 63, 205; p. 209) is advised before rupture occurs if the patient's general condition is good. Under these favorable conditions, the risk of fatality is under 2%.

Differing from aneurysms of the aorta which tend to rupture, aneurysms of the leg arteries are more likely to fill with clot and close off, blocking the flow of blood.

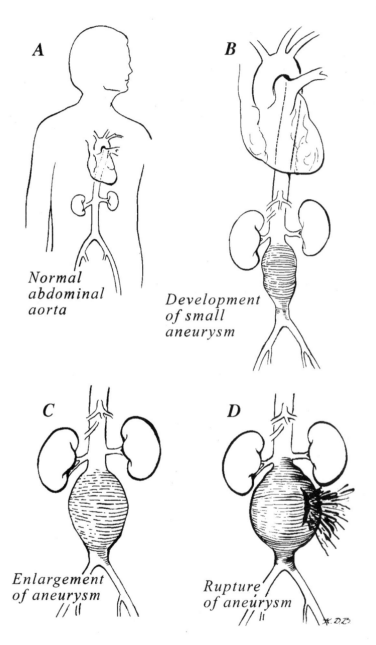

A

Normal abdominal aorta

B

Development of small aneurysm

C

Enlargement of aneurysm

D

Rupture of aneurysm

Figure 38 - Aneurysm development with progressive enlargement leading to rupture with massive hemorrhage.

Diagnosis

Diagnosis of the Two Main
Complications of
Hardening of the Arteries:
- Blockage of the Flow Channel
- Aneurysm Formation

- General Considerations 85-87
- Diagnosis of Blocked Arteries
  to the Heart 88-93
  to the Brain 94-101
  to the Kidneys 102-103
  to the Legs 104-107
- Diagnosis of Aneurysms 108-111

General Considerations

Proper treatment of a patient starts with finding out what is wrong. In many patients with atherosclerosis, the flow channel of critical arteries becomes **blocked**. In other patients, the wall may weaken and **bulge out** (aneurysm formation). Because these events can cause death, it is vital for doctors to find out if either or both of these threatening changes are present. In this section we discuss how these abnormalities may be diagnosed.

Blocked arteries are much more common than aneurysms and tend to occur where the flow channel divides, especially in the heart, neck, and legs (Fig. 39, p. 87. Such blockages cause pain in the muscles and nerves which are deprived of their blood supply. Aneurysms don't restrict blood flow and seldom cause pain until they rupture. Aneurysms develop most often in the big artery in the abdomen, the aorta, beginning about an inch below where the arteries to the kidneys arise (pp. 109-111). If aneurysms can be felt, they are easily diagnosed by their broad, strong pulsations. On the other hand, blocked arteries from atherosclerosis and clots have little or no pulsation.

If narrowing of the arterial channel is marked, it severely reduces the flow of blood to the tissues and causes a threatening decrease in the supply of oxygen, water, nutrients, and other chemicals to the cells. The symptoms and changes that become evident depend upon which organ or body part is deprived of its blood supply.

Blockage of the arteries that supply the *heart* is diagnosed by the patient's symptoms and by special studies that include:
1. Recording the electrical activity of the heart *[electrocardiogram* (ECG)] at rest and with exercise *(treadmill,* Fig. 40, p. 91)*, both early and late after a blockage, and by various blood tests in the early period.

2. Determining if calcification is present in the coronary wall by ultrafast computed tomography *(heart scan)*. If it is, hardening is proven. The scan shows hard plaques (Fig. 35, p. 75) but not soft ones (Fig. 34, p. 74). A high calcium score, however, indicates a high number of both types because they accompany each other.
3. Performing cineangiograms after injecting dye into the coronary arteries to show blockages (Fig. 41A, p. 93).

Blockage of the arteries that supply the *brain* is diagnosed by symptoms, presence of *murmurs* and *thrills* along the course of these vessels in the neck (Fig. 42, p. 95), and by reflected sound wave (Fig. 46, p. 101) and arteriogram (Fig. 45, p. 99) studies that show the arterial flow channels. Murmurs and thrills are caused by turbulence (chaotic, swirling flow) of the blood as it suddenly exits from a site of narrowing into a much larger channel. In the case of a murmur, the turbulence shakes the wall sufficiently hard that the vibrations can be *heard* with the aid of a stethoscope (Fig. 43, p. 97). In the case of a thrill, the turbulence shakes the tissues so hard that the vibrations can be *felt* by placing a finger lightly on the skin over the artery.

Blockage of the arteries that supply the *kidneys* is diagnosed by reflected sound wave (ultrasound) studies and arteriograms. The significance of such blockages can be assessed by the amount of *renin* in the blood. The more a kidney's blood supply is reduced, the more renin it secretes. The more renin, the tighter the little arteries throughout the body constrict, and the higher the blood pressure rises.

Blockage of the arteries that supply the *legs* is diagnosed by symptoms, appearance of the feet (both elevated and hanging down), exercise capacity, pulse quality, presence of murmurs and thrills at rest and after exercise, leg blood pressures at different levels, ultrasound studies, and arteriograms.

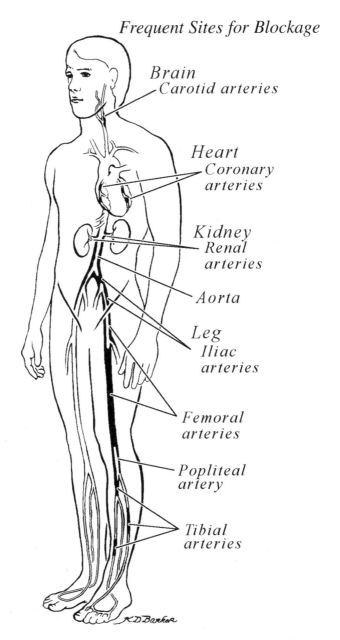

Frequent Sites for Blockage

Brain
Carotid arteries

Heart
Coronary
arteries

Kidney
Renal
arteries

Aorta

Leg
Iliac
arteries

Femoral
arteries

Popliteal
artery

Tibial
arteries

Figure 39 - Common locations of arterial blockages due to hardening of the arteries (inner wall) and clot formation.

Diagnosis of Blocked Arteries to the Heart

In years past, doctors thought that coronary heart disease was primarily a condition of men. Today, we know that this is not true. Coronary heart disease is just as common in women as it is in men, but on average it occurs about 10 years later. The reason for this delay appears to be the protective effect of estrogens (hormones secreted primarily by the ovaries) in premenopausal women. Like men, more women die of heart disease than from any other cause, especially if they smoke.

After menopause, lack of estrogens appears to accelerate the development of atherosclerosis. But the question is still unanswered, *"Does estrogen replacement therapy (ERT) reduce this tendency?"* ERT relieves menopausal symptoms and decreases the loss of bone substance (osteoporosis) in post-menopausal women. ERT, however, increases the risk of uterine and breast cancer. But taking progesterone, another ovarian hormone, with the ERT reduces the uterine, but not breast, cancer risk. ERT may not be advisable for women with a family and/or personal history of breast cancer. Instead, non-hormonal synthetic medications which protect the bones without increasing the risk of cancer may be used. If these issues are pertinent to you, please speak to your physician. Recent studies suggest that the weak estrogens found in plants called *phytoestrogens* may be effective without increasing the risk of cancer. Soybean phytoestrogens have shown some promise in this regard.

*About 950,000 people died of heart and artery diseases due to **atherosclerosis and clots** in the United States last year.* This total exceeded the deaths due to *cancer, infections*, and *accidents* combined. Of this number, about 450,000 died as a consequence of sudden blockage of vital coronary arteries, due most often to rupture of small, soft plaques with lipid cores (Fig. 34, p. 74). About half had no prior symptoms.

Sudden blockage of a vital atherosclerotic coronary artery by clot formation usually causes the heart muscle it supplied with blood to die because of lack of oxygen and nutrients. In lay terms, this event is called a "heart attack" or medically, a *myocardial infarction* or an "MI" for short.

During a heart attack, the patient often experiences severe chest pain/pressure and becomes pale, sweaty, cold, and clammy. Early in the attack, the deprived muscle, though dying, is still alive. At this point, **every minute counts!** If clot dissolving drugs can be given intravenously within the first hour after the pain begins, these remarkable medications can dissolve the clot that has formed over a ruptured or ulcerated plaque, restore the circulation, and save most (or even all) of the threatened heart muscle.

People who develop severe chest pain should call for help immediately (911 in nearly all areas of the United States) so that if they are having a heart attack, the medics can make the diagnosis quickly and begin treatment rapidly. Prompt action is often the difference between life and death.

As you can see, the diagnosis "heart attack" has become a true medical emergency because so much can be corrected by emergency treatment. Today, many patients are given clot dissolving drugs on the way to the hospital in Medic 1 emergency transport and treatment vehicles. In many cardiac treatment centers, patients received within the critical first hours are taken directly to the heart laboratory where cardiologists perform special studies and treatments, often balloon dilation procedures (frequently with stents) to maintain the flow channel. These will be discussed later.

Millions of people experience chest pain due to an *insufficient* supply of red blood to their hearts. Most feel pain only when the heart's need for oxygen and nutrients increases, as for example, during exercise, after eating, or in the midst of an emotional upset. This pain, called **angina** is most commonly felt in the pectoral region over the heart. The medical term for this is *angina pectoris*. Angina may also occur in the neck, jaw, shoulders, arms, and back. In addition, some patients feel *suffocating pressure,* as if an elephant were standing on their chests.

Strangely, some patients (especially women) with severe restriction of their coronary blood supply experience little or no angina. Instead, they *tire easily* because their hearts, which are short of oxygen and nutrients, can't pump enough blood to meet the body's needs. These patients, in fact, are in greater danger of sudden death from their hearts stopping than are those patients who, when warned by angina that the heart muscle needs more blood supply, stop their activities, place a nitroglycerine tablet under their tongue to dilate their coronary arteries, and wait for the pain to disappear.

The physician begins the evaluation of a patient who has had chest pains by asking questions about both this specific complaint and the background medical history, performing a physical examination, and ordering appropriate laboratory tests, including an electrocardiogram. Should these investigations suggest heart disease, the physician may send the patient to a heart specialist (cardiologist) at that point.

The cardiologist may order an *echocardiogram* and, for some patients, a *heart scan*. If the scan shows calcium in the walls of the coronary arteries, atherosclerosis (hardening) is proven. Nothing else causes this to occur.

Echocardiographic studies involve sending *sound waves* into the heart which echo back and are processed to give motion picture-like recordings of the heart's contracting ability, chamber size, wall thickness, and valve function. This study may be done at rest, during exercise, and after exercise.

The cardiologist may then decide to do a *treadmill* or *stress* test to observe the effects of progressive exercise on the patient's blood pressure, pulse rate, electrocardiogram, and symptoms. In this test, the patient walks in place on a moving surface at increasing rates and grades for specific time periods.

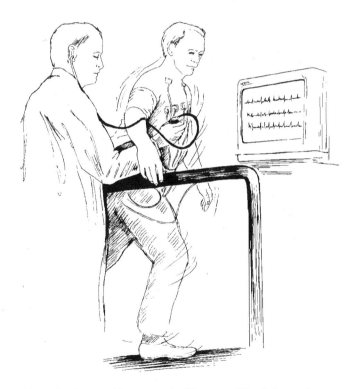

Figure 40 - Patient taking treadmill test. Physician observes patient and measures blood pressure during test.

If threatening changes occur during the test, such as a marked fall in the blood pressure; an irregular, slow, or fast pulse; major alterations in the shape of the ECG tracing; or the patient develops severe angina, weakness, or shortness of breath, the cardiologist will stop the test and note the elapsed time to when these changes began.

After termination of the test, the cardiologist observes the patient and his/her ECG and blood pressure, noting the time required for any stress-induced abnormalities to disappear.

Should the patient develop angina of lesser extent during the procedure that does not require stopping the test, the patient tells the cardiologist when it starts, how the pain progresses, and how long it lasts into the rest period.

If the treadmill test reveals findings suggestive of serious coronary heart disease (ECG changes indicative of a severe lack of blood supply to the heart and/or the early occurrence of marked angina), the cardiologist will probably next perform *coronary arteriograms* (cineangiograms) -- high speed x-rays of the arteries of the heart performed after injecting dye into them -- to show any blockages of the flow channels that may be present. Such obstructions may be assumed to be atherosclerotic thickenings of the inner wall which are often made worse by clots on their diseased flow surfaces.

Coronary arteriograms are performed by inserting a long, slender, hollow tube *(catheter)* into the big artery at the groin and advancing it upward into the arteries of the heart (Fig. 64, p. 207). The cardiologist then injects dye through the catheter and takes motion picture x-rays of the passage of this fluid through the coronary arteries. These films reveal any obstructions in the coronaries which block the circulation of blood to the heart muscle (Fig. 41A, p. 93).

After completing the studies, the cardiologist diagnoses whether the patient has coronary disease and, if so, what is the best treatment for it. This latter decision is often reached in consultation with a heart surgeon.

Operations are advised for patients who have severe angina that can't be relieved by medical treatment and/or have arteriograms which show life-threatening blockages (Fig. 41A, p. 93). Some patients are best treated by cardiologists who dilate the blocked coronary arteries with tiny balloons attached to the ends of long, slender catheters by a procedure called *balloon angioplasty* (Figs. 41B, 64-67; pp. 93, 207, 210, 211, 214). Other patients are best treated by surgeons who open the chest and implant *bypass grafts* (Figs. 69, 71-76; pp. 216, 218-223) that carry blood around the blockages.

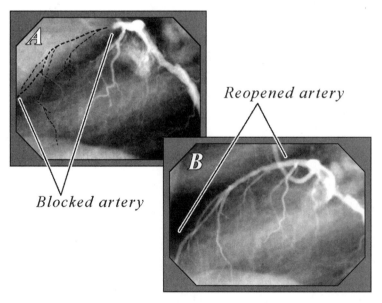

Figure 41 - Coronary cineangiograms (arteriograms) showing (A) acute blockage of upper portion of anterior descending branch of left coronary artery and (B) blood flow restored in this artery by emergency balloon angioplasty.

Diagnosis of Blocked Arteries to the Brain

Two pairs of arteries supply the brain, the *common carotids* and the *vertebrals* (Fig. 42, p. 95). The common carotids are about 3/8 inch in diameter and run upward, one on each side in the front part of the neck to carry blood to the brain and head. Each artery divides into two vessels at the level of the angle of the jaw. One vessel is named the *internal carotid artery* because it goes inside the skull to supply the eye and the front and middle parts of the brain on its side. The other vessel is called the *external carotid artery* because it runs outside the skull to supply the face, mouth, tongue, ear, and scalp on the same side. The division point of the common carotid arteries and the first inch of the internal carotid arteries are the sites most frequently afflicted by atherosclerosis.

The two *vertebral arteries* are the other pair of vessels that supply the brain. These arteries are about 1/4 inch in diameter and run upward, one on each side deep in the front of the neck. They pass through an opening in the side part of the upper six backbone segments in the neck and enter the skull where they unite to form the *basilar artery* which supplies the base and the back part of both sides of the brain. These vessels are less often involved by atherosclerosis than the carotid arteries.

When the blood supply to an area of the brain is blocked, its vital cells will be damaged or killed, causing loss of function. This condition, called a "stroke" or "brain attack," is caused either by fragments *(emboli)* of platelet clumps, clots, or cholesterol debris that are carried by the blood into the brain where they block vessels and shut off the blood supply; by *clots* which form in atherosclerotic brain arteries; or by *hemorrhages* from rupture of arteries that supply the brain. When a stroke occurs, the degree of brain function that is lost depends on what part of the brain is affected, how much is damaged or destroyed, and the effect that this injury has on the rest of the brain.

The stroke victim may be paralyzed on one side, and, in addition, be unable to feel, speak, see, swallow, smell, comprehend, perceive, or understand conversation. These and other deficits may occur in any combination and vary in all grades of severity. The loss of function may be temporary or permanent. Generally, the worse the initial deficit, the less the chance of regaining the lost function.

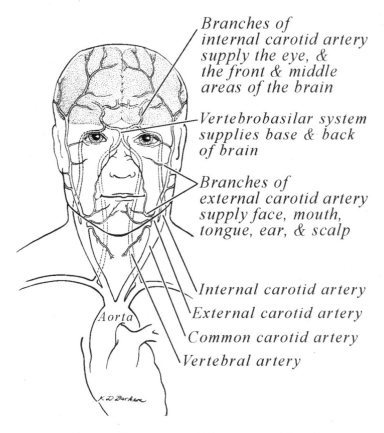

Branches of internal carotid artery supply the eye, & the front & middle areas of the brain

Vertebrobasilar system supplies base & back of brain

Branches of external carotid artery supply face, mouth, tongue, ear, & scalp

Internal carotid artery

External carotid artery

Common carotid artery

Vertebral artery

Aorta

Figure 42 - Arteries of the Brain and Head

As with a heart attack, strokes occur when vital cells lose their blood supply and die from lack of oxygen. *Dead brain cells cannot be replaced. They are gone forever.* Hence, **prevention** of strokes, rather than treatment of their disastrous consequences, is our **primary goal.**

About 50% of all strokes occur because atherosclerosis causes the inner portion of the wall of the common carotid arteries at their division point in the neck near the angle of the jaw to thicken and the surface that the blood flows over to become ragged and ulcerated, predisposing to platelet aggregation, clot formation, and embolization (Fig. 33, p. 71).

Platelets stick to these diseased surfaces like flies to honey. These adherent platelets become activated (sticky) and attract other platelets which stick to them and become activated. These newly activated platelets attract still more platelets which in turn stick to them and activate, etc., etc. This aggregation cascade leads to the formation of fragile clumps of platelets that project into the blood path where small fragments can easily break off. When this happens, these particles (emboli) are carried by the blood into the brain where they plug up little arteries and shut off the blood supply to the localized areas nourished by these vessels.

Fortunately, most of these platelet fragments break up within a minute or two because the lining cells of the arteries where they lodge secrete powerful chemicals which cause the platelets to lose their stickiness and separate. As this happens, the circulation returns and the stroke-like symptoms disappear quickly (Fig. 33, p. 71). But if the fragments are large, do not break up, or do so too late, the stroke persists.

Also, when the carotid artery is severely narrowed, there is danger that the blood in the tiny flow channel that remains will clot and close the channel off completely. If that happens, brain cells will likely die quickly from lack of oxygen and cause a *permanent stroke*. Severe strokes usually cripple patients for long periods before they kill them.

Fortunately, these threatening atherosclerotic changes in the carotid arteries can often be diagnosed while there is still time to prevent them from causing a stroke. *Two* easy *clues* make this possible. The **first** is the presence of *murmurs* which can be heard near the angle of the jaw with a stethoscope (Fig. 43, below). Murmurs are vibratory noises created by the turbulence produced when a column of blood jets suddenly from a narrowed channel into a large one where the flow is slower. In general, the smaller the narrowed channel becomes, the faster the blood flows through it.

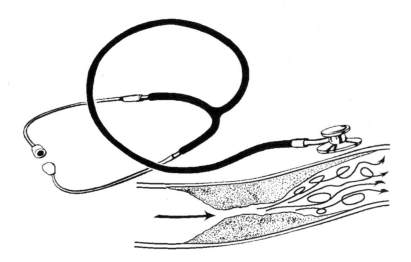

Figure 43 - A stethoscope is a listening device used in this case by the physician to hear murmurs (vibratory noises) generated by turbulent blood flow in the internal carotid artery just beyond a site of severe stenosis (narrowing).

The **second** clue which suggests that there is atherosclerotic disease in the carotid arteries is the history of one or more brief, stroke-like episodes called *transient ischemic attacks* (TIAs). This term refers to a temporary loss of function due to a momentary interruption of circulation to a small part of the brain (Fig. 33, p. 71; Fig. 44, below). The TIA may cause a brief loss of vision; sensation; the ability to speak, write, hold a glass, or walk; and many more types of deficits. TIAs get better quickly because the emboli (which cause these attacks) break up rapidly and allow the circulation to resume.

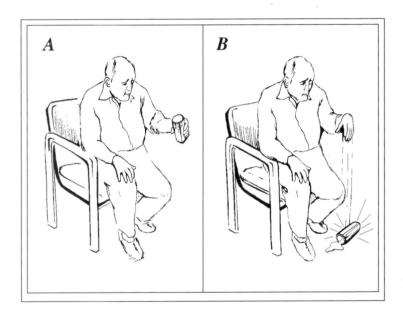

Figure 44 - This man drops the glass because a small platelet embolus to the right side of the brain has caused sudden weakness of his left hand. The left hand is affected because the right side of the brain controls the left side of the body and vice versa. If the embolus breaks up quickly and allows the circulation to resume, the weakness of the left hand will disappear rapidly. In that case, the episode is called a transient ischemic attack (TIA).

Patients having TIAs are at significant risk to develop a permanent stroke in the near future. Because of this, they should contact their physicians promptly or go to the emergency room of the nearest hospital. Unless their general condition is very poor, all patients who have had a clear-cut TIA should have further studies to determine if additional treatment is required. Until recently, this meant having x-rays of the arteries supplying the brain after injecting dye into them (Fig. 45, below).

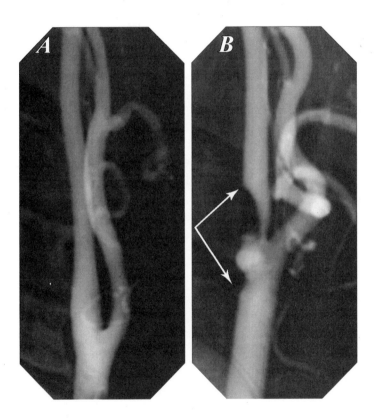

Figure 45 - (A) Normal right carotid arteriogram. (B) Abnormal right carotid arteriogram showing severe stenosis and ulceration involving the origin and first portion of the internal carotid artery. Extent of area involved shown by arrows.

Now, many patients who have suffered a TIA will only have
ultrasound studies, usually referred to as "Doppler" or
"Duplex" studies (Fig. 46, p. 101), instead of carotid
arteriograms because they are also highly accurate and, in
addition, have no risk, are painless, and cost much less than
x-ray studies -- about $300 versus $3,000.

The patient goes to a vascular laboratory where a technician
performs the ultrasound examination by passing a probe
along the skin over the carotid arteries. This probe generates
sound waves at a frequency of a few million per second that
are directed inward toward the underlying artery. These
waves are reflected back from the carotid wall and processed
to create an accurate image of the flow channel. But, if
calcification is present in the wall, the image is obscured.

The technician also uses the reflected sound waves to
measure the speed of the red blood cells as they flow through
the channel. The red blood cells flow faster as the channel
becomes smaller. This velocity measurement is an accurate
indicator of the caliber (size) of the arterial flow channel.
Ultrasound studies represent a major advance in the diagnosis
of vascular diseases, especially blockages.

If either ultrasound or arteriogram studies show severe
narrowing of the flow channel of an artery going to the brain,
surgery is usually advisable, especially if the patient has had
transient, stroke-like symptoms. The surgeon opens the
artery; removes the thick, diseased inner wall; and sutures the
normal outer wall back together to restore a full flow channel
that has a smooth, clot-resistant surface for the passage of
blood (Fig. 79, p. 229). Most patients who undergo this
operation are discharged home the next day.

Carotid Ultrasound Study

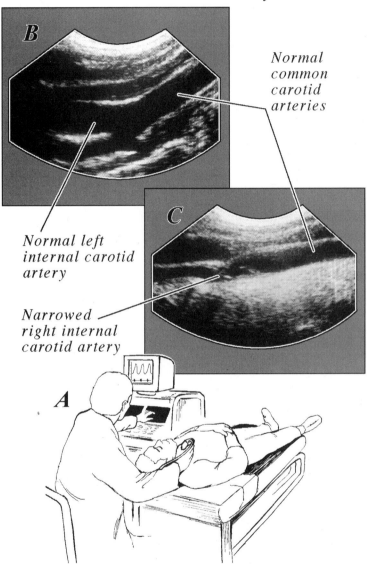

Normal common carotid arteries

Normal left internal carotid artery

Narrowed right internal carotid artery

Figure 46 - (A) Patient undergoing carotid duplex ultrasound studies. (B) Normal left carotid ultrasound findings. (C) Abnormal right carotid ultrasound findings showing plaque formation with severe narrowing in first portion of the internal carotid artery.

Diagnosis of Blocked Arteries to the Kidneys

The kidneys *filter* the blood and *excrete* a yellow fluid called *urine*. If the kidneys are unable to do their job adequately, waste products, water, and minerals (especially potassium) build up in the blood to the degree that they may poison the body and cause death. Also, since the kidneys make a hormone, *erythropoietin,* which stimulates the bone marrow to produce red blood cells, kidney failure causes anemia, too.

Severe blockage of the arterial blood supply to a kidney may lead to very high blood pressure (which responds poorly to drugs) and to impaired function and decreased size of the deprived kidney.

When a patient is found to have high blood pressure which cannot be controlled satisfactorily by medications, ultrasound studies and renal arteriograms may be advisable to determine if there is blockage of the blood flow to one or both kidneys (Fig. 47, p. 103). When there is a severe narrowing of a *renal* (kidney) artery, the flow of blood to that kidney is decreased. This causes the kidney to secrete more of the high blood pressure chemical called *renin*. This chemical reacts with other chemicals in the blood to form a compound which causes the small arteries throughout the body to constrict. It is the constriction of these vessels that causes the blood pressure to rise to very high levels.

Severely elevated blood pressure due to increased secretion of renin or to other abnormalities can make the heart work so hard that it fails. High blood pressure also makes the patient more prone to brain hemorrhage. It may impair vision, too. In addition, if there is blockage of only one renal artery, the high blood pressure can severely injure the "normal" kidney. Though high blood pressure due to decreased blood flow to one or both kidneys is infrequent, it must be carefully searched for in patients with severe hypertension who are resistant to medications. High blood pressure due to this cause can be corrected by balloon angioplasty (dilation and stent placement, Fig. 80, p. 231) or vascular surgery (removal of the thick, diseased inner wall or placement of a bypass graft to the open artery beyond the blockage, Fig. 79, p. 229 and Fig. 81, p. 232). The secretion of renin by a deprived kidney decreases when its blood flow is restored.

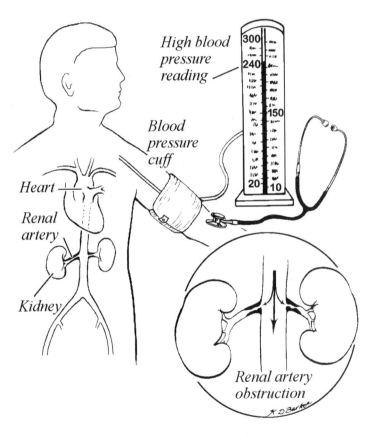

Figure 47 - Severe blockage of the blood supply to a kidney may cause very high blood pressure that responds poorly to medications.

Diagnosis of Blocked Arteries to the Legs

When the supply of red blood to a legs decreases, the changes
that develop depend on the severity of the blockage. The first
symptom is known medically as *intermittent claudication* (p.
286). This means an aching pain which develops in muscles
(most commonly those of the calf) that don't receive an
adequate supply of red blood during exercise. The pain
develops because the extra blood the muscles need to remove
the lactic acid that forms during exercise can't be supplied to
them by blocked, atherosclerotic arteries. The quicker the
onset of pain and the more severe it is, the longer the pain
takes to disappear. Resting the muscles allows the blood flow
time to catch up and relieve the pain.

If the reduction of blood supply is mild, muscle pain doesn't
occur until one has walked several blocks rapidly or climbed
several flights of stairs quickly. If the flow reduction is
moderate, muscle cramping occurs after walking two to three
blocks or going up a flight or two of stairs. If the reduction is
severe, muscle cramping occurs after walking half a block or
climbing a few stairs. Finally, if the flow reduction is critical,
severe cramping occurs after taking a few short steps.

When the reduction of circulation to a leg reaches this
advanced stage, other symptoms and findings appear. Severe
pain now develops in the foot within an hour or two after the
patient goes to bed. This agonizing symptom, called *rest
pain,* occurs because the blood pressure in the foot falls when
the patient lies down. The force of gravity, which helps blood
reach the foot in the upright position, is lost when the patient
lies flat in bed. This loss of gravitational pressure further
reduces the already critically reduced flow of red blood to the
sensory nerves of the foot and causes deep throbbing pain
which forces the patient to try and get some relief by sitting

in a chair or standing up. But the pain returns soon after the sleep-starved patient lies down again to try and get a little rest. Fortunately, bypass graft surgery can relieve the suffering and save the limbs of many of these patients.

If physical and Doppler (p. 100) findings suggest that arterial blockages are the reason why the patient is unable to work, can't enjoy reasonable activity, has rest pain, can't sleep, and/or has impending or actual *ulceration* of the toes, foot, or heel, a surgeon or radiologist will perform arteriograms (Figs. 48-50) to show which arteries have normal-sized flow channels and which have narrowed or closed ones.

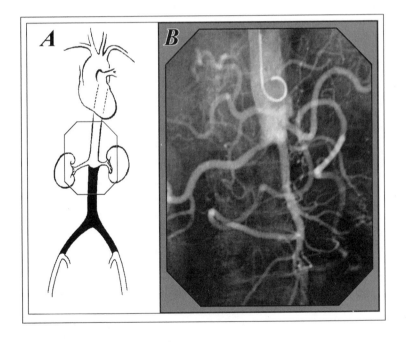

Figure 48 - (A) Drawing showing blocked aorta and common iliac arteries in abdomen. (B) Aortogram showing same thing with blockage of flow of red blood to pelvis and legs.

This information enables the surgeon to decide if it's possible to restore circulation to the limb. Patients with rest pain have such severe lack of circulation that the skin of their feet, especially of the toes, becomes pale, cold, and prone to break down and form *ulcers*. At this advanced stage, if the circulation can't be increased, *gangrene* with more tissue death, ulceration, and spreading infection is a constant threat. If this happens, the leg may have to be amputated to save the patient's life.

Fortunately, advances in foot care and surgical techniques have greatly reduced the need for amputations. Placement of long blood vessel grafts constructed of the patient's own veins is an effective way to increase the blood supply to the lower leg, even if the graft must extend all the way from the big artery at the groin to a small artery in the foot (Fig. 93, p. 247).

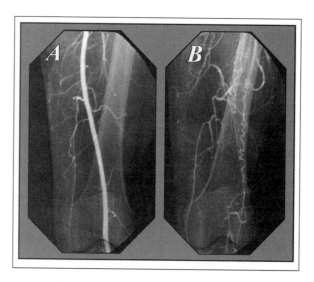

Figure 49 - Arteriograms showing (A) normal arteries in thigh and at knee and (B) blockage of these arteries with marked reduction of the supply of red blood to lower leg and foot.

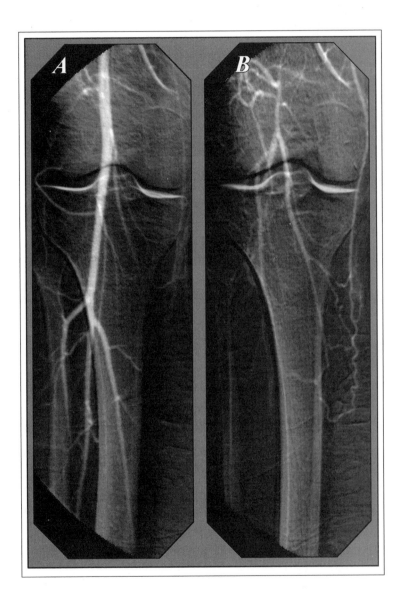

Figure 50 - Arteriograms showing (A) normal arteries at knee and in lower leg and (B) blockage of these arteries with severe reduction of the supply of red blood to lower leg and foot.

Diagnosis of Aneurysms

Aneurysms almost never give warning until they begin to rupture. Then the risk of surgery becomes very high. Patients with ruptured abdominal aortic aneurysms are often near death when they are brought to the hospital -- pale with low blood pressure and a painful, swollen abdomen.

Aneurysms due to atherosclerosis develop most often in the *aorta,* the body's largest artery, which emerges from the heart, arches up, slants to the left and extends backwards to descend through the posterior part of the chest (thorax) near the midline to continue into the abdomen. In the abdomen, the aorta reaches the midline at the level of the navel and divides into the right and left common iliac arteries which descend to supply the pelvis and legs below. *Aneurysms develop most often in the abdominal aorta, beginning about an inch below where the arteries to the kidneys arise.* Most are lined by clots. Fewer aneurysms occur in the thoracic aorta and even fewer occur in the arteries of the legs.

An unruptured aneurysm in the abdomen is seldom painful. It may be noticed incidentally by the patient who, one day, is surprised to feel a pulsating mass in the mid-part of his or her abdomen. More frequently, the pulsation will be detected by the patient's physician during a routine physical examination (Fig. 51). Often, flecks of calcium in the wall of the aneurysm will outline its presence on an x-ray of the abdomen taken for some other reason.

Usually, an aneurysm of the aorta in the chest will be suggested by a "shadow" discovered on an x-ray. Further studies of the types shown on pages 110, 111, which show abdominal aneurysms, are usually required to see if the "shadow" is an aneurysm or another type of abnormality.

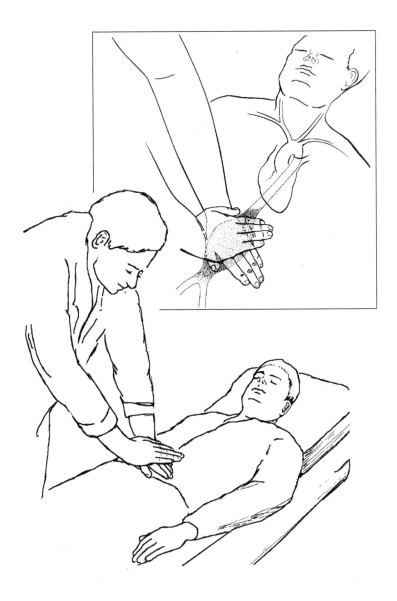

Figure 51 - Physician may diagnose an aneurysm of the abdominal aorta by feeling its prominent pulsation.

Years ago, *aortograms* were the best way to gain additional information about the aorta. This is no longer so because CAT scans (Computed Axial Tomography) and *MRI studies* (Magnetic Resonance Imaging) are safe, technological wonders which make precise diagnosis of aneurysms easy. Ultrasound studies of the abdominal aorta, though less precise, are also safe and cost much less than any of the other methods.

If the patient's general condition permits, the proper treatment for an aneurysm of the abdominal aorta is to replace it with a synthetic aortic graft, usually one made of Dacron fabric.

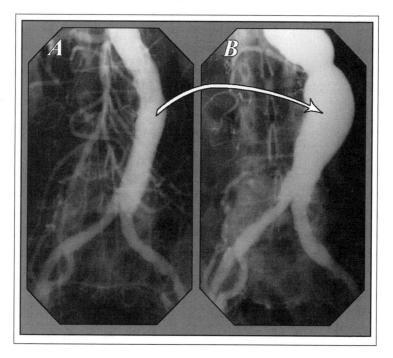

Figure 52 - (A) Aortogram showing elongated abdominal aorta of normal caliber. (B) Aortogram in this same patient six years later showing that this vessel has developed into a bilobed aneurysm.

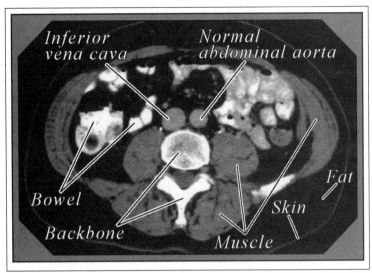

Figure 53 - CAT scan shows cross-section of abdomen revealing normal-sized abdominal aorta. (Note that the aorta is smaller than the inferior vena cava).

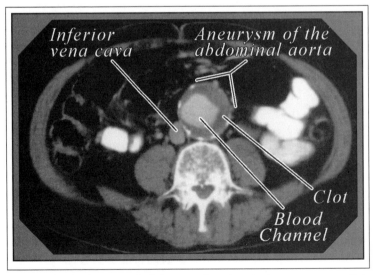

Figure 54 - CAT scan of abdomen showing large aneurysm of the abdominal aorta with considerable clot formation.

Section III:

Prevention

Prevention of Atherosclerosis and
Its Complications by
How We Live Our Lives

- Introduction 113-115
- Smoking -- *Deadly Foe* 116-135
- **The Better Life Diet**© -- *True Friend* 136-160

    Introduction 136
    Nutritional Basis* 137-152
    Meal Plan** 153-160

- Exercise -- *Essential Ally of Better Life Diet* 161-187
- Stress -- *Potential Killer* 188-189

* with Robert H. Knopp, MD

** by Anna Martin, BS, and Evette M. Hackman, PhD, RD

Introduction

I believe that most heart attacks and strokes; nearly all cases of lung cancer and emphysema; and most cases of type 2 diabetes (p. 279, 280), blindness, kidney failure, and lower extremity amputation can be prevented. Sound impossible? Far from it. Here's a **5 point strategy that will work** for you -- don't smoke and avoid inhaling other people's smoke, eat a heart-healthy diet, exercise regularly, achieve and maintain a healthful weight, and control your adverse responses to life's daily challenges. This is good health at a bargain you can't afford to turn down.

There's little disagreement that it's how we live, day by day and hour by hour -- more than anything else -- that influences how *long* we will live and how *well* we will live.

As we age, the quality and healthfulness of our lives become even more important to us. We need to decide today what we want our tomorrows to be **before it's too late to make a difference**.

Having a heart attack at age 39, coronary bypass surgery at 40 and again at 48, a blocked artery in one leg at 50, a bypass graft to that leg at 51, a blocked artery in the other leg at 53, a bypass to this leg at 54, repeat operations on both legs from ages 55 through 57 to remove clots from the grafts and restore blood flow to the legs, the loss of one leg at 58, a stroke at 60, loss of the other leg at 62, carotid artery surgery at 63, and another heart attack at 65 -- with a painful death a year later after several anguishing months of worsening congestive heart failure is *not* the way any of us wish to live or die.

Further, the life-time medical expenses for such a person could easily exceed $1 million. Instead of such a painful and costly experience, all of us would prefer to remain *healthy* until our time to depart arrives in our mid-eighties or beyond. There is wisdom in learning how to prevent atherosclerosis and associated clot formation instead of learning how to be a "good patient." My goal is to help you gain this preventive wisdom.

But even if you already have symptoms of cardiovascular disease, don't despair because there's an excellent chance you can turn things around by redirecting how you live your life, starting today.

Be joyful because what you will learn in this section and the next one about heart-healthy (fit) living could save your life and the lives of many of your loved ones.

While there will always be need for excellent heart surgery, I believe its role in a few years will be primarily that of a backup for failed prevention. I predict that such failures will become infrequent in the future for those who choose to follow the evolving directives of heart-healthy (fit) living. In addition, those who require surgery will come to better appreciate that they also need the best of prevention (pp. 112-199) for the rest of their lives to attain maximum benefit and avoid repeat operations.

If we, as a society, do not take disease prevention more seriously, medical costs will continue to rise and could bankrupt our health care system within a few years.

While medical care has properly come to be accepted as a right in our society, *accepting disease prevention* as a concomitant *binding obligation of citizenship has lagged far behind*. This medical disconnect must be corrected.

The challenge before us is clear. Each of us must recognize that the maintenance of our own health is a serious *personal* responsibility -- a responsibility that we owe to ourselves, our families, and our *nation*.

Risks and Consequences

Lifestyle Risk Factors & Physiological Results	Leads to...	Consequences
Smoking • Increases fibrinogen • Makes platelets sticky • Raises homocysteine (p.197) • Constricts small arteries • Increases blood pressure • Decreases oxygen in blood • Increases cancer potential • Destroys lung elasticity	**Development of** **Type 2 Diabetes**	Heart attacks Sudden cardiac death
Diet high in low-fiber carbs, refined sugar, saturated fat, *trans* fatty acids, and calories* • Raises LDL cholesterol, triglycerides, and insulin • Increases weight -- fat • Increases cancer potential	**Hypertension** **Hardening of the**	Congrestive heart failure Strokes Decreased walking capacity
Too little aerobic exercise • Drops HDL cholesterol • Increases fibrinogen • Makes platelets sticky • Increases weight -- fat	**arteries** **Clot**	Leg ulcers, gangrene, and amputations Blindness
Excess weight (obesity) • Lowers sensitivity to insulin • Raises glucose, insulin, LDL c, and triglycerides, • Reduces exercise ability • Promotes type 2 diabetes	**formation** **Tumor growth**	Kidney failure Aneurysms and hemorrhages Many cancers, esp. lung
Uncontrolled stress • Makes platelets sticky • Constricts small arteries • Increases blood pressure	**Emphysema**	Slow suffocation

*Figure 55 - Lifestyle choices which increase our risk of cardiovascular and other diseases. * See glossary for details.*

<u>Smoking</u> -- *Deadly Foe*

Unfortunately, addiction to smoking occurs before its tragic physical consequences become evident. This is why smokers, both men and women, have so much difficulty stopping. Their shortened lives rob them of precious years with their loved ones, and their loved ones of previous years with them.

These *disastrous* medical *consequences* of *smoking* are:
1. The accelerated development of **atherosclerosis** ("hardening of the arteries") that causes clot formation which leads to heart attacks, strokes, high blood pressure, decreased walking capacity, limb loss, blindness, kidney failure, and hemorrhage from ruptured aneurysms.
2. A greatly increased risk of many types of **cancer**, especially of the lung.
3. Progressive destruction of the elastic tissue in the lungs that leads to **emphysema** and slow suffocation.

Smoking overshadows *all* other major risk factors for development of atherosclerosis, including high blood pressure, obesity, diabetes, and blood-fat abnormalities. Even the tobacco industry now admits its products are addictive and deadly.

There's more. Mothers who smoke during pregnancy *harm* their babies. Stillbirths, premature births, low birth weight, and sudden death in the early months after birth (Sudden Infant Death Syndrome -- SIDS) are all more common when mothers smoke. And that's not all. The kidneys of some premature infants remain small and cause them to have high blood pressure as adults.

There are many more reasons why people who smoke now *should stop,* and why those who don't should *never start.*

More on Health Risks of Smoking

Shortened Life Expectancy: The risk of death from smoking varies directly with the *number of packs* and *length of time* one has smoked. The person who has been a two-pack-a-day smoker for 15 to 20 years *will die six to eight years sooner* than a nonsmoker. With these odds, why would anyone want to smoke? And there's much more.

Heart Disease: Smokers are *twice* as likely to have a heart attack and *five times* more likely to die from it than nonsmokers. Smoking decreases oxygen and increases blood pressure (p. 120).

Stroke: Smoking *doubles* the risk of stroke.

Decreased Walking Capacity and Limb Loss: Because smoking accelerates hardening of the inner arterial wall and predisposes this hardened wall to have clots form on it, the smoker is at risk for blockage of the circulation in many areas of the body. In the legs, such blockages may make walking very difficult. Lack of blood supply necessitates leg amputations in about 100,000 people yearly in the U.S. Limb loss is rare in people who don't smoke and don't have diabetes.

Lung Cancer: Cigarette smoking causes nearly all lung cancers in the U.S. Lung cancer is the leading cause of cancer deaths among both men and women. "Marlboro Men" and "Virginia Slims Women" *die early*. Lung cancer and cardiovascular disease cause 50% and 900% more deaths, respectively, in women than breast cancer!

Mouth Cancer: Smokers, tobacco chewers, and snuff users have about 10 times as many oral cancers as nonsmokers. Drinking alcoholic beverages increases this risk.

Cancer of Larynx: Smoking increases the risk of developing laryngeal cancer about *five times* that of nonsmokers.

Cancer of Esophagus: Cigarette, pipe, and cigar smoking *triple* the risk of developing this cancer. Drinking alcoholic beverages also increases the risk of developing this cancer.

Cancer of Pancreas: The risk of smokers developing this cancer is *double* that of nonsmokers.

Cancer of Colon: Smoking a pack of cigarettes a day for 10 years *doubles* the risk of developing this cancer.

Cancer of Bladder: Smokers have about a *seven times* greater risk of developing this cancer than nonsmokers.

Cancer of Breast: Over *half* of Caucasian-American women and about a *third* of African-American women carry a gene that slows the rate of detoxification of tobacco-related carcinogens. Among postmenopausal women with this gene, those who have smoked heavily at *any* point in their lives have *four times* the risk of breast cancer compared to those who have never smoked (JAMA, Nov 13, 1996).

Emphysema: Smoking causes nearly all cases of this deadly disease. The lungs lose their elasticity and become big, nonfunctioning airbags into which little air can be moved in or out. In the advanced stages of emphysema, the patients must sit up and struggle for each breath as they slowly suffocate.

Osteoporosis: Smoking causes early onset in women.

In view of the foregoing, smoking is clearly a dangerous, addictive habit that has no redeeming virtues. It's all bad and kills millions of people worldwide each year.

Dollar Costs of Smoking

The costs of smoking in the United States are huge:

- The retail sale of cigarettes and other tobacco products is about $50 billion a year, $1 billion of which is spent by children and adolescents.

- Health care costs attributable to cigarettes and other tobacco products are also about $50 billion a year.

The total annual cost of tobacco products and the consequences of their use in the United States is at least $100 billion. This figure does *not* include the cost of fires caused by smoking, or the increased cost of insurance premiums as a result of such fires. Nor does it include the cost of government subsidies to tobacco farmers. Just think of the good that this money could bring if it were used instead for purposes that would *benefit* people.

It's easy to understand why we must continue to urge those who smoke to stop, and those who don't smoke not to start. An encouraging fact is that today there are over 50 million ex-smokers in the U.S. (including 100,000 physicians).

But smoking by teenagers, especially girls -- many of whom do so in an effort to stay slim -- is increasing. An estimated 3,000 children and adolescents start smoking each day in the U.S. (about one million each year). It's not a coincidence that the tobacco industry has targeted this vulnerable group. Ninety percent of today's adult smokers started smoking *before* they reached the age of 20. Big tobacco's strategy is clear -- *addict them early!*

How Smoking Damages the Cardiovascular System

Cigarette smoking increases the heart's workload and, at the same time, prevents the heart from getting the oxygen it needs to do its work. This double "whammy" is comparable to living at 14,000 feet in the Andes Mountains and having to do twice as much work as at sea level. Not a good plan.

The **nicotine** and **carbon monoxide** in cigarette smoke attack the body simultaneously in two ways to cause major heart trouble. First, *nicotine* enters the blood and causes the tiny arteries throughout the body to constrict. This raises the blood pressure which increases the work of the heart and requires it to use more oxygen. Second, *carbon monoxide* enters the blood and combines with hemoglobin in the red blood cells. This reduces the ability of hemoglobin to carry oxygen to the cells, including those of the heart. The nicotine-carbon monoxide combination is deadly.

In addition to nicotine and carbon monoxide, there are many other toxic chemicals in cigarette smoke (p. 122), including millions of oxygen free radicals (pp. 197, 271) that are inhaled with each drag. These toxins damage the lining (endothelial) cells of arteries and the lining cells and elastic structure of the lungs. These injuries predispose the arteries to atherosclerosis ("hardening of the arteries") and the lungs to cancer and emphysema.

Nicotine and carbon monoxide are especially damaging because nicotine increases the workload of the heart while carbon monoxide decreases its oxygen supply. Smoking also increases clotting by making the platelets in the blood "stickier" and the level of fibrinogen higher.

Questions And Answers
About Smoking

Q. *Are people really smoking less? It seems as if everyone around me smokes.*

A. Seventy-five percent of American adults do not smoke. Furthermore, of these 150 million people, about 50 million are ex-smokers, 95% of whom quit on their own without professional help.

Q. *Tell me more about the risks of smoking.*

A. The risk of early (and painful) death increases in direct relation to the extent of smoking.

The average long-term, two-pack-a-day smoker will lose about 2,500 days of life. Since the value of even one day of living is beyond measure, the real price of smoking can't be calculated.

Q. *Any other reasons for quitting smoking?*

A. Yes! You'll have more energy, and you'll be able to breathe easier, too.

Your senses of taste and smell will return.

If you don't smoke, there's a good chance your children won't either.

Your breath, clothes, and home will smell better.

You'll have fewer colds and bouts with the flu, and

those you have will be less severe.

The children in your household will have fewer colds, respiratory problems, and ear infections.

Your nonsmoking spouse will not be at increased risk of developing coronary heart disease, lung cancer, and emphysema from inhaling your cigarette smoke. Show your true love by stopping!

Your home will be less likely to catch fire, and your insurance premiums will be lower.

You'll also save lots of money. For example, if a person starts smoking two packs of cigarettes a day at 15 years of age and continues doing so for 24 years, the total cost would be about $48,000. If that money had been invested in tax-free, 6%, zero-coupon municipal bonds instead of cigarettes, the worth of the bonds would be $111,000 at the end of that period. The net savings would be $159,000. A nice nest egg! And even nicer if you had bought stock in Microsoft "back then" when it was a real bargain.

Q. *Tell me about nicotine, tar, and carbon monoxide.*

A. The "high" you feel when you smoke is real. It comes from the nicotine in the cigarette smoke that increases your heart rate and blood pressure. This is how nicotine addicts its victims.

A one-pack-a-day smoker inhales about one cup of tar each year. This terrible material contains the bulk of the cancer-causing agents ("**carcinogens**") that are present in cigarette smoke.

Carbon monoxide is a colorless, odorless gas which is 640 times more concentrated in cigarette smoke than what is considered safe in our nation's industrial plants. This deadly gas combines with the hemoglobin in the red blood cells where it displaces a significant amount of oxygen, making it harder for the tissues to get the oxygen that they need. Carbon monoxide, along with nicotine, tars, and other chemicals in cigarette smoke, accelerates the development of atherosclerosis, cancer, and emphysema.

Q. *Are smokers sick more often than nonsmokers?*

A. Yes. The National Center for Health Statistics estimates that smokers spend an estimated 88 million extra days sick in bed each year than do nonsmokers.

Q. *What are the symptoms of lung cancer?*

A. They include persistent cough, blood in the sputum, lingering infection of the lungs, and pain in the chest. By the time such symptoms appear, the chance for cure of the cancer is very low.

Q. *What is the correlation between inhaling smoke and my personal health risk?*

A. The more you smoke, the more you inhale. Most smokers inhale even though they aren't aware of doing so. And the more you inhale, the greater your chances are of developing coronary heart disease, lung cancer, and emphysema.

Q. *How long does it take to put yourself at risk for accelerated coronary heart disease, lung cancer, and emphysema?*

A. Experts call it a "dose-related response." That means the more you smoke the more you're at risk.

Each cigarette you smoke does some harm; the day-by-day accumulation of this damage can cause disease to develop. A pack of cigarettes a day for 15 years -- one million drags -- will put you into the high-risk zone for coronary heart disease, cancer, and emphysema. This is Russian roulette with a vengeance. **It makes no sense for you or anyone.**

Q. *Are filter cigarettes, low-tar/low-nicotine cigarettes, pipes, or cigars safer?*

A. It was once believed that filter cigarettes were safer: after all, they were designed to help filter out some of the tar and the other chemicals in tobacco smoke. It is now known, however, that filters tend to concentrate the carbon monoxide in smoke, making these cigarettes **even more dangerous** than those they were meant to replace.

Studies show, too, that people who switch to low-tar/low-nicotine cigarettes often inhale more deeply and smoke more in order to compensate for the reduced nicotine.

Cigarette smokers who switch to a pipe or cigars are very likely to inhale. This keeps them at risk for the same diseases that cigarettes cause. **The deadly smoke is the same.**

Q. *Is the damage done by smoking reversible?*

A. Yes, to some degree. If a disease process due to smoking has not already begun, and the individual stops smoking for the next 10 years, his or her life expectancy after that period will be significantly improved. But there is less certainty about the extent of protection from lung cancer.

Also, those who quit smoking after having coronary bypass or other vascular surgery fare much better than those who don't quit.

Some harmful effects of smoking will begin to disappear soon after you stop. In weeks to months your senses of taste and smell will return, and your cough will go away. You'll feel less winded. Your circulation will improve. Your elevated blood pressure will drop, and your heart won't have to work as hard.

Remember, you can quit for good; over 50 million other Americans have.

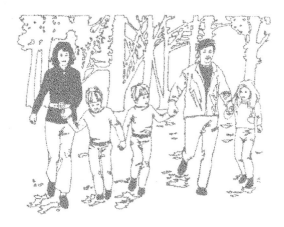

How To Quit

Ninety-five percent of the 50 million U.S. citizens who have quit smoking have done so without the aid of an organized smoking cessation program, according to the Department of Health and Human Services. An encouraging note.

The following suggestions for "kicking the habit" have been compiled from many sources and may be what you, your spouse, or your friends need to become ex-smokers.

Before You Quit

✔ Write down all the personal reasons you have for wanting to quit smoking (such as your health, doctor's advice, cough, smell of smoke in clothes, and cost). Read this list aloud each night before going to sleep, and read it aloud again each morning before you do anything else.

✔ *Think only of the benefits of quitting.* (Don't let yourself think about how difficult it might be and how many unsuccessful attempts you've made in the past.) Get excited about becoming an ex-smoker!

✔ Set your "Quit Day" for the near future. (Your child's birthday, the first day of spring, or an anniversary are possibilities, but don't delay.) Consider your "Quit Day" sacred once you have set it, and don't let anything or anyone change it.

✔ Incorporate other positive lifestyle changes into your life. (Start by having a good breakfast each morning, taking a 30-minute brisk walk every day, eating more fruits and vegetables, and going to bed on time.)

✔ Find a friend who wants to quit smoking with you. Talk it over and plan how you'll support each other after you've both quit.

✔ Consider switching to a brand of cigarettes you dislike or changing to a brand that's very low in tar and nicotine a few weeks before you quit. Both of these strategies will help decrease your addiction to nicotine. The second plan works *if* you don't smoke more cigarettes or inhale more deeply to increase the "kick."

✔ Stop buying cigarettes by the carton; only buy them one pack at a time. Wait until your pack is empty before you buy another one. Walk to where you buy them -- don't drive. *Make it difficult to get more.*

✔ Make yourself aware of each cigarette by smoking with the opposite hand and putting your cigarettes in an unfamiliar pocket to break the automatic reach.

✔ Reach for a glass of sparkling water or spicy vegetable juice for a "pick-me-up," instead of a cigarette.

✔ Don't empty your ashtrays. The rancid smell of burnt-out cigarettes and their repulsive sight will soon disgust you and strengthen your determination to stop smoking.

✔ Don't think of quitting smoking "forever." Take it the way recovering alcoholics do, ". . . *one day at a time.*"

✔ Allow yourself to smoke only in one place and don't do anything else while you do. Don't eat, drink, socialize, read, or watch TV while you smoke.

✔ Open your package of cigarettes and throw one cigarette away. When you buy another pack, open it and throw two away. The key is to keep the time between packs the same while you progressively adjust to longer and longer times between "smokes." The next pack, throw three away . . . and so on. You'll have increasingly longer periods of not smoking until you just stop completely by the 20th pack or sooner.

✔ Do things that require using your hands such as needlework, craft work, crossword puzzles, or even building an addition to your home.

✔ Reorganize your life to avoid situations that "call" for a cigarette. (Go for a walk after dinner instead of watching TV. Get up earlier to avoid morning hassles. If you drink coffee, stop. Switch to tea to break the coffee-cigarette habit. Keep sugarless gum handy in your car.)

✔ Ask your doctor about nicotine replacement medications -- nicotine gum, patches, and nasal spray. These diminish the short-term symptoms that may occur when you stop smoking. Also, ask about *Zyban*, a prescription medication that reduces the urge to smoke.

Once You Quit

✔ Keep sugarless gum and low-calorie, crunchy foods handy such as carrots, pickles, cloves, fresh ginger, apples, and celery.

✔ A few times a day during the first week after you quit take 10 deep breaths and hold the last one while you light a match and pretend it's a cigarette. Then blow it out, and crush the "dirty thing" in your ashtray which is full of snuffed-out, foul-smelling butts. Yes, smoking is a really miserable habit!

✔ Practice relaxation techniques to reduce tension and overcome the urge to smoke. For starters, try relaxing in a comfortable chair, breathing deeply, and thinking pleasant thoughts.

✔ If you feel a really threatening urge to smoke coming on, tell yourself, "I won't give in, not now, not ever!" If the desire keeps mounting, take a relaxing hot shower and finish with a cold rinse. Tell yourself, "I can do it. I'll never go back." Then drink a glass of cold water and you'll be okay again -- back in charge of your life.

✔ Never allow yourself to think: "Just this one time, it's okay to have a cigarette." *Total abstinence* is the key.

✔ Avoid social situations where smoking is allowed. Instead, go to exercise facilities because they don't allow smoking, and the activities there are good for you. A hard combination to beat.

✔ When you feel tense and frustrated and want a cigarette, go for a brisk walk and before long you'll be back in charge.

✔ After a week or so when you feel in control, throw away all your remaining cigarettes, matches, ashtrays, and lighters. (Don't store them; you'll *never* need them again. Think positive. Don't waver. **Remember, it's your life you're saving!**)

✔ On the day you quit, make plans to keep busy. Go to a movie, take a hike, go bike riding, go to dinner -- nonsmoking section, of course.

✔ Buy yourself something you've always wanted, or do something special to celebrate your "Quit Day."

✔ Go to the dentist and have your teeth cleaned of cigarette stains.

✔ Drink lots of water -- at least eight glasses a day. (Try sparkling or bottled water with lemon if you don't like tap water.)

✔ Avoid alcoholic drinks, coffee, and other beverages you once associated with cigarette smoking.

✔ As soon as you finish a meal, brush your teeth. It will help break the habit of reaching for a cigarette.

✔ If you must be where you'll be tempted to smoke, associate with the nonsmokers who are there.

✔ *Pay special attention to your appearance.*

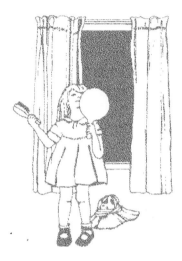

✔ Clean your clothes, sheets, blankets, pillows, draperies, and rugs to rid them of that musty, rancid smell of stale cigarette smoke.

✔ Whenever a new reason for stopping smoking flashes through your mind, write it down on your list of reasons why you'll never smoke again. Keep this expanding list on your bathroom mirror or refrigerator door where you will see it frequently.

✔ Ex-smokers relapse most often during times of boredom, frustration, anger, tension, loneliness, and worry. Have a battle plan to help you through these difficult times, such as exercising, reading, calling a friend, or saying a favorite prayer.

What To Expect After You Quit

The First 12 to 72 Hours After You Quit:

You will find that these early hours are the hardest and most critical times of your battle to free yourself from the addictive grip of nicotine. If you don't stop smoking and go through this early, painful period, you'll never win your freedom. Just stop and tell yourself, *"I'll be okay in a few days."*

During those early days you may experience shortness of breath, chest tightness, fatigue, insomnia, visual disturbances, sweating, nervousness, headaches, stomach pain, bowel upset, irritability, and an inability to concentrate.

It's important to understand that initial, unpleasant changes after quitting smoking are *temporary*. They are a result of your body adjusting to the absence of nicotine, a truly addictive drug. Maintaining a positive attitude, eating regularly, drinking plenty of water, getting extra exercise, and breathing in lots of fresh air will help you get through these difficult early days.

The First Month After You Quit:

After these first few days, you'll begin to notice some remarkable changes in your body. Your senses of taste and smell will gradually return, and if you have a smoker's cough, it will start to slowly disappear, too. Your head will feel clearer -- no more headaches or dizzy spells from cigarettes. You'll be able to breathe easier, and you'll have more energy. **You'll wonder why you ever started smoking, and why you didn't stop sooner.**

The Second and Third Months After You Quit:

Now, the worst is definitely behind you, but unexpectedly you may experience moments of intense desire for a smoke. The aroma of fresh cigarette smoke may continue to "smell good" for several months. Don't panic. You'll be okay. These feelings will disappear with more time.

Be forewarned. When you first quit smoking, you may enjoy considerable praise and support from your friends and family. But over time, their support will decrease even though you may still be struggling, one day at a time. Be ready for this possibility and hang in there.

The Fourth Month to the Fourth Year After You Quit:

After having apparently "won the battle," many fail here by falling into the old "one-can't-hurt" trap. Unfortunately, one cigarette can lead to another and in no time you could be "hooked" again. Don't give in. Ask yourself if the brief "fix" provided by that one cigarette could really be worth going through all the unpleasantness and agony of having to quit again. But if you should fall, don't despair. Get up and go on 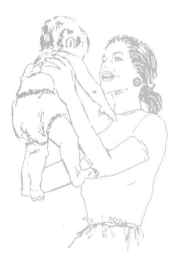 more determined than ever to win this battle for your life. Six to eight more years of happy living with your family and friends are surely **worth whatever effort it takes to permanently free yourself from this deadly addiction.**

But if you *do* succumb and have a cigarette, know that the nicotine you absorb from that *one* experience is not enough to get you *hooked* again. Don't lose control. Use the *fall* as a learning experience that will prepare you to overcome future temptations.

Some would-be ex-smokers fail because they light up in reaction to every type of crisis or undue stress that develops either at work or at home. They believe that a cigarette will aid and comfort them. The truth is, it won't. If you've recently quit smoking, decide now what you'll do instead of reaching for a cigarette when the going gets tough.

Note: Among ex-smokers who haven't smoked for five to nine years, one out of five still report an occasional craving for tobacco. It's addictive stuff, but you can beat it -- 50 million other Americans have. They are living proof that you, too, can win your freedom.

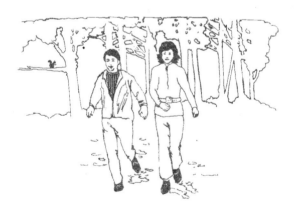

How to *Avoid* Gaining Weight
When You Quit Smoking

Studies have shown that only one-third of people who quit smoking gain weight and that this group on average gains less than 10 lbs. If you have recently stopped smoking, the following suggestions will help you control your weight.

- Weigh yourself several times a week.

- Read the nutrition and exercise sections (pp. 136-187), and follow their recommendations.

- Enjoy the **Better Life Diet** and get at least 30 minutes of brisk exercise every day to reduce stress, build muscles, and burn calories.

As part of a successful plan to stop smoking, some people find that "indulging" themselves a bit with an occasional special meal or tasty dessert during the first few months after quitting smoking helps them say "No" to the voice that says "Have just one, it won't hurt." They find that they can lose the few added pounds *later* when they are safely on their way to becoming a *permanent ex-smoker.*

Should you need additional help in your effort to stop smoking, please contact:

- The Hope Heart Institute: (206) 903-2254, Fax (206) 903-2244); email lsauvage@ hopeheart.org; http://www.drsauvage.com
- The American Heart Association: (your local listing).
- The American Cancer Society: (your local listing).
- The American Lung Association: (your local listing).

The Better Life Diet -- *True Friend*

Introduction

As a heart surgeon I saw the devastating results of heart disease on a daily basis for 33 years. That experience has focused my post-surgery career on how to best help people live long and youthful lives. Clearly, **prevention** is the way to do this -- *not more surgery*. The wise application of accurate, understandable information is the key.

Today, people are overwhelmed by the sheer mass of competing diets and claims. The *Pritikin* and *Ornish* diets advise about 80% of calories from carbohydrates, 10% from fats, and 10% from proteins. The *Atkins* diet advises almost no carbs initially while encouraging unlimited quantities of fats and proteins. The *Sugar Busters* diet avoids sugar. *The Omega Diet* focuses on types of fatty acids. The *American Heart Association* diet advises high-fiber carbohydrate intake with moderate fat restriction. The *Protein Power* and *Zone* diets advise high-protein consumption.

I have selected the best from these diets and combined this information with what I've learned in taking care of thousands of patients. The result is the **Better Life Diet©**.

As stated on page 113, I believe that most premature deaths from heart attacks and strokes; nearly all cases of lung cancer and emphysema; and the majority of cases of type 2 diabetes (p. 279, 280), blindness, kidney failure, and lower extremity amputation can be prevented.

Is this possible? Yes, if you don't smoke, follow the **Better Life Diet and Exercise Program,** attain and maintain a healthful weight, and minimize unhealthy emotional stress. By making this lifestyle become a reality, you will be empowered to achieve the long and youthful life you deserve. This is my goal for you!

The Better Life Diet *-- *True Friend*

*Nutritional Basis***

There are three basic types of food: **carbohydrates (carbs), fats,** and **proteins**. Carbs and proteins are calorie poor (four calories/gram). Fats are calorie rich (nine/gram). Among other actions, carbs provide energy and fiber. Fats make cell walls, brain matter, hormones, and energy. Proteins form enzymes, antibodies, hormones, building materials, hemoglobin, muscles, and energy.

The **Standard American Diet ("S.A.D.") causes many to die prematurely**. It has too many calories, too many low-fiber carbohydrates (white bread, mashed potatoes, french fries, and white rice), far too much refined sugar, too much saturated fat, and too many *trans* fatty acids. *In addition to their improper and excessive diet, most Americans don't exercise nearly enough.*

Standard American Diet

1. Too many calories

2. Too much
- Low-fiber carbohydrates
- Refined sugar
- Saturated fats
- *Trans* fatty acids

3. Too little
- High-fiber carbs (fruits, vegetables, and whole grains)
- Legumes (peas, beans, and lentils)
- Mono and omega-3 unsaturated oils
- Fish
- Skinless poultry
- Nuts and seeds
- nonfat/low-fat dairy products
- Low-fat meat
- Shellfish

Figure 56 - Some deficiencies of the Standard American Diet.

* With Robert H. Knopp, MD, Professor of Medicine and Director, Northwest Lipid Research Clinic of the University of Washington.
** We become what we eat. See Glossary for further information about carbohydrates, cholesterol, diabetes, fats, fiber, insulin, obesity, proteins, refined sugar, *trans* fatty acids, and vitamins.

Who doesn't look forward to sitting down with family and friends to enjoy a good meal? Though eating is pleasurable and necessary for life, we must control what we eat to live a long and healthy life. Our **Better Life Diet** does this. This diet is based on seven broad guidelines. It does not depend on detailed calorie counting. Enjoy this diet for life. Use it to lose or maintain weight as needed.

The Seven Guidelines of the Better Life Diet

To reduce obesity, type 2 diabetes (p. 279), kidney failure, cancer blindness, hypertension, atherosclerosis, clots, heart attacks, strokes, and limb loss, we advise these enjoyable guidelines:

1. **Eat plenty** of high-fiber carbohydrates, such as fresh fruits -- an apple a day is hard to beat; fresh vegetables; legumes (peas, beans, and lentils); whole-grain breads, cereals, and pastas; and whole grains, such as brown rice (pp. 283,284).
2. **Markedly restrict** low-fiber carbohydrates, such as white bread, mashed potatoes, french fries, and white rice (p. 284).
3. **Drastically restrict** refined sugar, white or brown (p. 140).
4. **Choose** protective fats, i.e., oils (e.g., monounsaturated types, such as olive and canola, and polyunsaturated omega-3 types, such as fish and flaxseed -- pp. 281-283).
5. **Severely restrict** saturated fats and *trans* fatty acids (p.142).
6. **Enjoy** proteins with little saturated fat (fish; skinless poultry; eggs - p. 146; legumes; nuts; seeds; nonfat/low-fat dairy products; *low-fat meat*, as lean beef, lamb, and center cut pork loin/chop or roast; and *shellfish*, as clams, oysters, mussels, crabs, shrimp, lobsters, and scallops.
7. **Drink** at least two quarts of water a day (8 glasses).

If you are significantly overweight, this balanced diet of high-fiber carbs (50% of calories), protective fats (30%), and low-saturated fat proteins (20%), when combined with a good exercise program (pp. 161-187), will autoregulate your weight over time to where you will feel and look your best and be able to stay that way.

Good Proteins - 20%

`4 cal/gm`

- Fish
- Skinless Poultry
- Eggs
- Legumes
- Nuts and Seeds
- Nonfat/low-fat Dairy
- Low-fat Meat
- Shellfish

Protective Fats - 30%

`9 cal/gm`

- 2/3 or more from mono and polyunsaturated (esp. omega-3) oils
- 1/3 or less from saturated fats and *trans* fatty acids

High-Fiber Carbohydrates - 50%

`4 cal/gm`

- Fresh Fruits
- Fresh Vegetables
- Legumes - - Peas, Beans, and Lentils
- Whole-Grain Breads, Cereals, and Pastas
- Whole Grains, such as Brown Rice, Whole Wheat, Oats, Barley, Bulgur, and Rye

*Figure 57 - Building Block Diagram of the 50-30-20 **Better Life Diet** reflects the origin of approximately 50% of calories from carbohydrates (mainly high-fiber varieties), about 30% from fats (mainly protective mono and polyunsaturated omega-3 types), and about 20% from proteins (mainly those categories that have little association with saturated fats). Also pages 145,146.*

More people are dieting. Yet more people are obese! Why? Too many diets fail to distinguish between high, low, and non-fiber (sugar - p. 144) carbs; saturated (bad) and unsaturated (good) fats; and high-bad and low-bad fat protein sources. Bad fats; *trans* fatty acids; and *excesses* of low-fiber carbs, refined sugar, and proteins (which are converted into saturated fat) decrease the liver's ability to remove LDL cholesterol (pp. 142, 276, 282) from the blood. High blood levels of this chemical cause heart attacks and strokes.

To reduce LDL cholesterol, one must exercise and restrict whole milk, cream, butter, and foods made with them, such as high-fat cheeses, rich ice creams, pies, and cakes; poultry skin; fatty red meats; low-fiber carbs; refined sugar; and commercially processed, hydrogenated foods (p. 142), such as most margarines, crackers, cookies, candies, chips, dips, doughnuts, and desserts.

The average American eats **150 lbs.** of refined sugar/year, yielding 760 calories/day -- 38% of the calories in a 2,000 calorie diet. Sugar (sucrose) contains no fiber, minerals, phytochemicals (from plants), or vitamins -- only calories. Soda pop and watered-down juice drinks are full of sugar -- 10 teaspoons in a popular cola (ten times the total glucose in all the blood in your body).

Real people in the real world need the **enjoyable meal plan** of *The Better Life Diet* (pp. 153-160). This diet provides about **50% of calories from carbs**, mainly from high-fiber varieties (few from low-fiber carbs or refined sugar); **30% from fats**, mainly protective (liquid) types (*i.e.,* oils); and **20% from proteins**, mainly those with little associated saturated fat. This tasty, filling, healthful, and practical high-fiber diet makes eating a pleasure, not a punishment.

Fiber, the portion of carbohydrates that our bodies can't digest, *is good for us because it slows digestion, reduces insulin secretion, minimizes changes in blood glucose, and decreases appetite.* (Imagine the "hype" for a drug that had these attributes!)

Most carb calories should come from fruits, vegetables, legumes, whole grains and their products (but few from white bread, mashed potatoes, fries, white rice, and refined sugar -- p. 138).

Most fat calories should come from oils, *i.e.,* liquid (unsaturated) fats. Monounsaturated oils, such as olive, canola, avocado, and peanut oils are good for us. Some polyunsaturated omega-3 oils , such as fish, flaxseed, and walnut oils are even better (*see* p. 281, 282 for omega-3 guidelines). Calories from saturated fats and *trans* fatty acids should not exceed 10% of the total calories you consume in a day. Saturated fats (such as butter) and hydrogenated oils (such as in many margarines) are soft solids at room temperature (p. 142). Excesses of these "hard" fats are far worse for our arteries than is enjoying a second egg for breakfast.

Most protein calories should come from fish (p. 146), *skinless* poultry; eggs; legumes; nuts; seeds; nonfat/low-fat dairy products; low-fat meat, such as lean beef, lamb, and center cut pork loin/chop or roast; and shellfish (p. 138). Few protein calories should come from *unskinned* poultry, *expensive* red meats (e.g., filet mignon), or *whole milk* since they have excess saturated fat.

This high-fiber carbohydrate, unsaturated fat (oil), and low-sat.-fat protein **Better Life Diet** protects our arteries from hardening and clotting. This diet prevents marked rises and falls in blood glucose and related insulin secretion that cause recurring waves of profound fatigue, uncontrollable hunger, and excessive eating, all of which lead to obesity, type 2 diabetes, and hypertension -- powerful risk factors for coronary heart disease (pp. 279,285,286).

The **Better Life Diet combined with enjoyable daily exercise** (p. 167) is optimal for the vast majority of people who wish to look and feel their best. For the few whose livers can't remove LDL cholesterol from their blood (a "gene" problem, p. 199), we advise physician-prescribed LDL-lowering medications ("statins" and niacin) in addition to our **Diet and Exercise Program**.

Foods High in Saturated Fats
and
Foods High in *Trans* Fatty Acids

Restrict calories from saturated fats and *trans* fatty acids to not more than 10% of total calories consumed daily.

Saturated Fats:

1. Whole and even reduced-fat milk (p. 143), and foods made with these types of milk, such as high-fat cheeses.
2. Cream (sour/table/whipped), and foods made with cream, including rich ice creams.
3. Butter and foods made with butter.
4. Poultry skin (contains most of the fat in poultry).
5. Fatty (marbled) red meats.
6. Canned meats.
7. Processed meats such as bacon, lunchmeats (e.g., bologna, pastrami, and salami), and sausage.
8. Lard and foods made with lard.
9. Coconut, palm, and palm kernel oils, and foods made with these saturated tropical oils.

Trans Fatty Acids:*

1. Vegetable shortenings and foods made with them.
2. Many margarines (p. 282) and foods made with them.
3. Commercially processed foods made with hydrogenated "oils"* such as crackers, cookies, cakes, candies, chips, dips, doughnuts, pies, other pastries, and peanut butter.

* Many margarines and most commercially processed foods (pp. 146, 153 for healthy peanut butter) contain hydrogenated soybean or other oils. Hydrogenation changes these oils into products that are soft solids at room temperature. This change occurs because hydrogen is added to the molecular structure of the oils, producing *trans* fatty acids. These acids are as dangerous as saturated fats because they also bind LDL receptors in the liver and impede the removal of LDL cholesterol from the blood. This effect of hydrogenation causes the LDL cholesterol levels in the blood to rise. Such elevations become dangerous when they reach 130 mg/dL (an average value -- pp. 276, 277, 282, 289).

The **Better Life Diet** uses only nonfat or low-fat milk. There are four designations of milk according to its fat content: whole, reduced-fat, low-fat, and nonfat. Whole milk contains too much saturated fat and so does reduced-fat milk. A cup (8 ounces) of whole milk has 150 calories and 5 grams of saturated fat (4%); a cup of reduced-fat milk has 120 calories and 3 grams of saturated fat (2%); a cup of low-fat milk has 100 calories and 1.5 grams of saturated fat (1%); and a cup of nonfat milk has 80 calories and no fat. People who are lactose-intolerant can usually digest four ounces (1/2 cup) of milk at a meal or can drink calcium-fortified soy milk.

The areas of the **Better Life Diet** Building Block Diagram (Fig. 57, p. 139) accurately reflect the origin of calories from carbs (50% - 4 cal/gm), fats (30% - 9 cal/gm), and proteins (20% - 4 cal/gm). For a 2,000 calorie daily intake, this means 250 grams of carbs, 67 grams of fat, and 100 grams of protein.

The **Better Life Diet** emphasizes high-fiber carbohydrates, unsaturated fats (oils), and good proteins (p. 138). While this diet doesn't eliminate any foods, it markedly restricts low-fiber carbohydrates (such as, white bread, mashed potatoes, french fries, and white rice), drastically restricts refined sugar (white or brown), and severely restricts saturated fats and *trans* fatty acids.

This tasty diet assures an adequate supply of calories (energy), building materials, fiber, minerals, phytochemicals, vitamins, and water. Also, the **Better Life Diet** markedly reduces the glucose stimulus for excess insulin secretion which further protects against obesity, type 2 diabetes, blindness, kidney failure, atherosclerosis, clots, high blood pressure, heart attacks, strokes, and limb loss.

The **Better Life Diet** provides 30% of total calories from fat, mainly from unsaturated liquid types, such as olive, canola, nut, soybean, fish, and flaxseed oils. Even though these oils protect our arteries, they, like all fats, are so high in calories (9 calories/gram) that they must be taken in moderation. The **Better Life Diet** also requires a marked reduction in low-fiber carbohydrates and a drastic reduction in refined sugar (pp. 140, 274, 289 and below*).

----

* **Sucrose (table sugar) is digested rapidly into glucose and fructose. This drives the blood *glucose* up, which suppresses hunger and *causes the pancreas to secrete insulin*. Glucose falls. Hunger returns. When more sugar is eaten, the cycle repeats. *Fats and proteins have little effect on insulin*. Vegetables and whole grains (because of their high fiber content) and fruits (because of their fiber and type of sugar -- fructose) convert more slowly into glucose and stimulate less insulin secretion. Milk sugar (lactose) causes a lesser insulin response, too. All these foods have lower *glycemic indices* (p. 284) than glucose alone. Insulin enables all the cells of the body to use glucose for energy and causes excess glucose to be stored as glycogen until its limited storage sites are filled (p. 274). Then insulin converts any excess glucose that remains into saturated fat and prevents it from being used for energy (p. 150).**

The up-and-down sugar-insulin relation fans the appetite; fats and proteins suppress it. **Eating sugar and low-fiber carbs throughout the day stimulates the pancreas to secrete large amounts of insulin which quickly changes any glucose that can't be stored as glycogen into saturated fat. Such a diet creates an overload of this *bad* fat. But, markedly restricting low-fiber carbs and drastically restricting refined sugar in the diet lowers insulin secretion and enables stored fat to be used for energy when the glycogen stores are exhausted. Making this source of energy available helps correct obesity and helps prevent type 2 diabetes (pp. 279,280), kidney failure, hardened arteries, clots, hypertension, blindness, heart attacks, strokes, and limb loss.**

The Better Life Diet *all but deletes* table sugar, standard soft drinks (soda pop), sugary "juice" drinks with less than 50% "fruit juice", jams, jellies, cakes, candies, pies, ice creams, and most other desserts. By following the Better Life Diet, the average daily consumption of refined sugar in a 2,000 calorie diet can be easily reduced from about 760 calories to 80 calories (pp. 153-160), decreasing the blood glucose and insulin levels.

We can learn much about the influence of diet on health from studies of **select population groups**. For example:

Japanese emigrants to the U.S. who adopt our American diet (p. 137) develop an increased incidence of obesity, type 2 diabetes, coronary heart disease, and breast and colon cancer. This suggests that the traditional native Japanese diet which is high in high-fiber carbs and low in low-fiber carbs, refined sugar, saturated fats and *trans* fatty acids is protective against these conditions.

Deaths from breast and colon cancer are uncommon in **countries where the diet is low in saturated (animal) fat.**

Seventh-Day Adventists in the U.S. who restrict or avoid tobacco and meat have less coronary heart disease, lung cancer, and emphysema than the general population.

The Five Basic Food Groups

Comparable Caloric Servings for the
Different Food Groups
and
Number of Servings Required

Fruits
- 1 whole medium-sized fruit like an apple, pear, or peach (about 1 cup - 8 oz.)
- 1/4 cup dried fruit
- 1/2 cup canned fruit
- 1/2 to 3/4 cup unsweetened fruit juice

Vegetables & Legumes
- 1/2 cup cooked vegetables or legumes
- 1/2 cup raw chopped vegetables
- 1 cup raw leafy vegetables
- 1/2 to 3/4 cup vegetable juice

Breads, Cereals & Pastas (whole grain)
- 1 slice bread
- 1 medium muffin
- 1/2 small bagel or English muffin
- 4 small crackers
- 1 small tortilla
- 1/2 cup cooked cereal
- 1/2 cup cooked rice
- 1/2 cup cooked pasta

Milk & Milk Products
- 1 cup (8 oz.) low-fat milk or yogurt
- 1 slice low-fat cheddar cheese, 1/8" thick (1 oz.)
- 1 cup of low-fat cottage cheese

Meat & Meat Alternatives
- 3 oz. (size of a deck of cards) cooked *lean* meat, skinless poultry, or fish*
- 2 eggs**
- 7 oz. tofu
- 1 cup cooked legumes (dried beans or peas)
- 1/2 cup nuts or seeds
- 2 tablespoons (32 grams - a little more than 1 oz.) of natural peanut butter - **not hydrogenated**

* **The omega-3 oils in fatty, cold-water fish, especially salmon, tuna, sardines, trout, and mackerel are protective of our arteries. Next to lignan-rich flaxseed oil, fish oil contains the largest quantity of the valuable omega-3 fatty acids. Eat fish often (p. 281, 282).**

** **One to two eggs per day are good for you unless you are diabetic or have high blood values for LDL cholesterol and/or triglycerides. In that case we recommend that you limit eggs to 3 to 4/week. The liver makes about 3000 mg. of cholesterol/day. One egg contains about 200 mg. of cholesterol.**

Number of Servings Required

	Children, Women, Older Adults	Teen Girls, Active Women, Most Men	Teen Boys, Active Men*
Calorie Level[1]	About 1,600	About 2,200	About 2,800
Fruit Group	2	3	4
Vegetable and Legume Group	3	4	5
Bread, Cereal & Pasta Group	6	9	11
Milk & Milk Products Group[2]	2 to 4	3 to 5	4 to 6
Meat & Meat Alternatives Group	2	3	4
Grams of fat[3]	**53**	**73**	**93**

* Girls and women of comparable size, muscle mass, and activity level need the same number of calories as their male counterparts.

1. **Servings of the major food groups** required at different calorie levels for the **Better Life Diet** (pp. 138,139).

2. **Teens, young adults, pregnant women, nursing women, and women concerned about preventing osteoporosis** need the higher number of servings (or additional calcium from alternative sources).

3. **Number of grams of fat when 30% of daily calories are from fat sources.**

20 Ways to Lower
the Saturated Fat and *Trans* Fatty Acid
Content of Your Diet

1. Microwave, bake, broil (on rack), poach, braise, or stir-fry foods instead of pan or griddle frying them when possible.

2. Use nonstick olive or canola cooking spray and a nonstick frying pan instead of adding butter or margarine.

3. Cook bacon and other fatty breakfast meats well, and then press them firmly between absorbent paper towels to remove as much of the remaining fat as possible.

4. Buy red meat with the least fat. "Prime" grade has the most fat, "choice" less, and "select" still less.

5. Purchase hamburger that is labeled "extra lean" and cook it well under the broiler to remove even more saturated fat.

6. Trim away all visible fat from meat before cooking and eating. This step can remove hundreds of calories.

7. Reduce the amount of saturated fat in canned meats, broths, and stews by chilling the cans before opening them. This causes the fat to rise to the top and solidify, making it easy to skim off.

8. Prepare foods in which the fat cooks into the liquid (stews, boiled meats, and soup stock) a day ahead of time. Then chill the food and remove the saturated fat which rises to the top and hardens.

9. Broil meats on a rack rather than frying them because the juices and liquified fat will collect in the pan below.

10. Defat these drippings if you make gravy with them by adding ice cubes to the drippings. This causes the fat to solidify and cling to the ice cubes, enabling it to be easily removed.

11. Limit meat to three 3-ounce servings (size of a deck of cards) of lean varieties a week. Eat more fish, poultry (without skin), eggs (p. 146), legumes (peas, beans and lentils), nuts, seeds, nonfat/low-fat dairy foods, and shellfish (pp. 138,139).

12. Remove the skin before cooking poultry because most of the fat is in, or just under, the skin.

13. Eat turkey year-round, not just on Thanksgiving Day. The white meat eaten without the skin is best. It's lowest in fat.

14. Substitute mustard, ketchup, relish, mayonnaise, or salsa for butter or margarine in sandwiches.

15. Enjoy low-fat yogurt or nonfat sour cream on potatoes instead of butter or margarine (p. 282).

16. Choose canola oil for low- or high-heat cooking but olive oil only for the lower-heat ranges. Both are protective of our arteries. In addition, olive oil is especially good for salads and bread dipping. Flaxseed oil also protects our arteries. Though excellent for salads, this oil is too heat-sensitive for cooking.

17. Switch from whole milk or reduced-fat milk to low-fat or nonfat milk. Your taste preference will change in several weeks. Once you've become accustomed to nonfat milk, whole milk will taste unbearably thick and fatty.

18. Remember that an "imitation" product may have as much or more "bad" fat as the natural product if it is based on hydrogenated and/or tropical oils. Read the labels.

19. Pick the softer margarines because they have fewer *trans* fatty acids. Squeezable margarines have the least, tub types intermediate amounts, and stick margarines have the most of these "bad" fatty acids (pp. 142, 193, 282, 283, 290).

20. Select low-saturated fat ("light," "diet," or "part-nonfat") cheeses and salad dressings instead of the high-fat varieties.

Basics for Weight Control

While the body can store little extra carbs or protein, it can store almost limitless quantities of fat in the fat cells (adipocytes) of the fatty (adipose) tissue. Too much or too little fat is harmful. The right amount is 15-20% of a man's normal weight and 20-25% of a woman's. *All digestible carbs are converted into glucose.* Glucose stimulates the pancreas to secrete insulin, which rapidly converts any excess glucose (that not needed for energy and unable to be stored as glycogen) into saturated fat. Less than a pound of glycogen can be stored in the entire body, 1/3 in the liver and 2/3 in the muscles. High insulin levels block the use of fat for energy. As a result, a one way street is created -- fat in, no fat out.

But if low-fiber carbohydrates are markedly restricted and refined sugar is drastically reduced, weight reduction becomes relatively easy for most people - - if combined with a consistent, sensible exercise program (p. 167). This dietary restriction reduces the insulin level in the blood and enables the excess fat stores to be used for the energy needs of the body (p. 144). At the same time, exercise increases energy needs and speeds fat loss (p. 185). The **Better Life Diet and Exercise Program** is also well-suited for people with Syndrome X (p. 290).

To lose excess stored fat, we must consume it for energy. There is no other way, short of surgery (pp. 186, 187) to eliminate excess fat. To burn a pound of stored fat per week requires a negative caloric balance of about 600 calories per day. You can achieve this by decreasing your caloric intake (diet) and/or increasing your caloric output (exercise). To lose that pound/week, you must burn about 67 grams (9 calories/gram) or about 2.3 ounces of your excess stored fat every day to supply these calories which your body is using in excess of the amount you are eating. To lose weight faster -- eat less, exercise more, or do both. If you follow the five cardinal rules for healthy living (pp. 191-195) you'll become fit and be pleased.

Achieving and Maintaining Your Ideal Weight

Each person has an "ideal" weight that is best for his or her physiological makeup. When you follow the **Better Life Diet and Exercise Program**, your body will self-regulate over weeks to months (depending on need) to your proper weight range and remain there so long as you stay with the program (p. 152).

In the U.S., about 30% of adults and 12% of children are obese.* Obesity decreases cellular sensitivity to insulin, predisposes to type 2 diabetes (p. 279), and produces biochemical changes that cause arteries to harden and wear out (p. 272). Losing even a few pounds of excess fat and *keeping these pounds off is important.*

People become overweight because they eat too much and don't exercise enough. Crash diets *aren't* the answer. In the almost inevitable relapses that follow such diets, much more fat is added than muscle. The result is a fatter and weaker person who wonders what went wrong. **Losing this excess fat and adding muscle** requires a new way of living built around eating the right foods in the proper amounts and exercising *every* day (pp. 138,161-187).

Weight Loss Strategy

If you are overweight, there is a pleasant solution for your problem: *start the* **Better Life Diet and Exercise Program**. Over the next month you will develop a taste for this appetizing diet, attain a full capacity for the sensible, aerobic exercise routine (2 miles of brisk walking daily and 5 minutes of slow, repetitive - - reach for the sky or horizon - - lifting of 3 - 6 lb. handweights each morning and evening), and lose about 1 lb./week. If you wish to lose weight faster, increase your walking over the next month to four miles daily and don't eat *any* low-fiber carbs or refined sugar while adhering to the rest of your dietary and exercise plan.

* Body Mass Index of 30 and above -- (BMI = $\frac{\text{weight in lbs. x 703}}{\text{height in inches}^2}$)

On this accelerated program you will lose 1/2 to 1 pound *more* per week. When you reach your target weight, continue the **Better Life Diet** (pp. 138, 139, 191-195) **and Exercise** (pp. 151, 166, 167, 174, 175, 191-194) **Program** at a level where you will look and feel your best indefinitely.

Excess weight is saturated fat waiting to be used for energy. The *two basic requirements* to begin the fat burning process are:
1. **Eat fewer calories** than you use (eat less, exercise more).
2. **Decrease your insulin secretion** by severely restricting the low-fiber carbs and refined sugar in your diet. This reduction enables fat stores to be used for energy (pp. 138,139,144,150), preventing obesity and type 2 diabetes.

Combining these two dietary strategies with a good exercise program develops muscle and burns the excess stored fat.

Weight Gain Strategy
In the U.S., far more people need to lose rather than gain weight. But being very thin is dangerous, too. **Emaciated people** have minimal stored fat. If they become ill and unable to eat, they **must burn their muscles (protein) for energy**. Such people have no reserves and their immune systems become depleted rapidly.

If you need to gain a significant amount of weight, calories are what count. Eat four, five, or even six meals a day that appeal to your taste. If this approach doesn't work, contact your physician promptly. Unexplained major weight loss must be investigated.

A note about alcohol: High consumption harms the heart, brain, and liver of both men and women. But in moderation, alcohol may have some protective action against coronary heart disease. Women are more sensitive to alcohol than men. Even in moderation, alcohol intake in women is associated with some increased risk of breast cancer. The reason for this is unknown.

The Better Life Diet -- *True Friend*
Seven day Meal Plan
with Nutritional Analysis

Anna Martin, BS, and *Evette M. Hackman*, PhD, RD,
Department of Consumer Science, Seattle Pacific University

Some comments about following **The Better Life Diet menu**:

• Eating well should progressively become a way of life for you. Your body and mind will respond positively to the changes you are making. Please note, however, that fiber intake should be increased gradually in order to avoid the unpleasant side effects of a sudden "fiber overload," for example: gas, bloating, and abdominal cramping.

• As you look at the nutrition information for each day, you can see that eating is not an exact science. There will be some variation in your daily food intake and calorie distribution. Your goal should be to meet **The Better Life Diet's** 50/30/20 caloric percentages for carbohydrates, fats, and proteins, respectively, by the week's end rather than on a daily basis. Also, this meal plan has been constructed for a 2000 calorie diet. Your needs may be smaller or larger (p. 147).

• Under the daily nutrition information, the total sugar count includes naturally occurring sugars (found in fruits, some vegetables, and milk -- p. 144) as well as added refined sugar. For each day of the menu, the refined sugar comprises no more than 10% of the total sugar count. Also, for each day of the menu, the combined saturated fatty acids (SFAs) and *trans* fatty acids (TFAs) comprise no more than 10% of the total calories.

• Nuts & Nut Butters: Nutritionally, the best nuts to choose are peanuts, almonds, and walnuts, but do not feel restricted to these choices. When shopping for natural nut butters, look at the ingredient list. *Peanut butter*, for example, should read peanuts and salt only (no hydrogenation). Other varieties of nut butters are available at natural food stores, including cashew, hazelnut, macadamia, soy "nut", and more.

• **These menus were designed as guidelines to help you learn how to eat well and enjoy! Please view them as examples rather than the rule.** Here are some other valuable resources to help you on your way:

1. *The Art of Nutritional Cooking, 2nd edition* by Michael Baskette and Eleanor Mainella. Upper Saddle River, NJ: Prentice-Hall, Inc.; 1999.

2. *Sunset Quick, Light, and Healthy* by the editors of Sunset Books. Menlo Park, CA: Sunset Publishing Corporation;1996.

3. *Cooking Light Magazine* by Doug Crichton, editor. Learn more on the web at www.cookinglight.com.

• Throughout the menu, when no beverage is specified, you may choose to enjoy *water*, coffee, tea, diet soda, or other **non-caloric** drink.

B = breakfast   **L** = lunch   **Sn** = snack   **D** = dinner

DAY 1 (vegetarian)

B: French Toast
>   2 pieces wheat berry bread
>   2 whole eggs
>   cinnamon to taste
>   topped with:
>>   2 teaspoons (tsp.) butter (about 8 grams)
>>   1/2 cup fresh berries (4 oz.)
>   1/2 cup fruit juice
>   1 cup (8 oz.) nonfat light yogurt

L: Garden Burger
>   1 vegetable burger
>   1 whole grain hamburger bun topped with:
>>   1 tsp. each: catsup, honey mustard, mayonnaise
>>   1/2 oz. reduced fat cheese
>>   2-3 slices of tomato
>>   2-3 leaves of spinach
>   1 oz. blue corn tortilla chips
>   1/4 cup salsa
>   1 cup nonfat milk

Sn: Fruit Smoothie
>   3 oz. soft tofu
>   1/2 mango
>   1/2 banana, frozen
>   1/2 cup guava nectar
>   1 packet Equal® sweetener
>   2 tablespoons (Tbsp.) nuts of choice

> The *Better Life Diet* meets the nutritional needs for the vast majority of Americans in a tasteful, satisfying, and healthy manner (pp. 136-152).

D: Curried Lentil Soup
>   1 cup (8 oz.) water with vegetable broth added
>   1/2 cup dry lentils
>   1/8 cup each: diced potato, carrot, celery, onion
>   1/8 tsp. each: ginger, garlic, curry powder
>   1 1/2 tsp. olive oil
>   1 medium slice wheat loaf bread oven-baked with
>>   1/2 oz. reduced fat cheese, shredded
>   1 cup spiced coffee (add dash of cinnamon & nutmeg before brewing)
>   1 small almond biscotti, 3-inch size

Nutrition Information: Day 1
Total Cal: 2043; % Carb: 53, % Fat: 28, % Pro: 19, SFAs+TFAs: 8.7%;
>   Total Fiber: 46 grams (g); Total Sugars: 100 g (≤ 10% is refined).

DAY 2

B: Cold Cereal
1 cup Cheerios®
1/2 cup nonfat milk
1 banana, sliced
1/2 cup nonfat cottage cheese topped with
1 Tbsp. (about 1/2 oz.) each: raisins, sunflower seeds
1 cup fruit juice

L: Fish Soft Taco
2 oz. halibut dipped in lime juice and bread crumbs, then broil
cabbage slaw: 1/2 cup cabbage, 2 tsp. mayonnaise, pepper & rice
vinegar to taste
1 large garlic & herb flavored tortilla
2 Tbsp. salsa
fresh cilantro to taste
1/2 cup egg drop soup
8 oz. nonfat light yogurt
2 persimmons

> **The *Better Life Diet* supplies
> all the daily requirements for
> vitamins and minerals.***

Sn: Hummus with Pita
1/2 wheat pita pocket, cut into 4 wedges
top each wedge with:
2 Tbsp. hummus
1 each: tomato slice, cucumber slice, fresh mint leaf

D: Grilled Vegetable & Ham Sandwich
1 medium sized whole wheat hoagie roll
1 oz. ham, deli meat
1 cup grilled vegetables: eggplant, squash, tomatoes, mushrooms,
bell peppers
1 oz. Havarti cheese spread on roll:
1 Tbsp. plain nonfat yogurt
1/2 tsp. Dijon mustard
1-2 cloves roasted garlic
1 tsp. olive oil (about 1/6 oz.)
1/2 cup nonfat cottage cheese
1 cup watermelon slush, blend together:
1 cup watermelon cubes, frozen
1 packet Equal® sweetener
1 1/2 Tbsp. lemonade, frozen concentrate

Nutrition Information: Day 2
Total Cal: 1983; % Carb: 53, % Fat: 26, % Pro: 22, SFAs+TFAs: 6%;
Total Fiber: 36 g; Total Sugars: 143 g (≤ 10% is refined).

* For additional protection, we advise selected supplements (pp. 162, 197).

DAY 3

B: Vegetable Omelet
>   2 whole eggs
>   1 cup diced vegetables: tomatoes, bell peppers, mushrooms,
>   onions
>   1/2 oz. reduced fat cheese
>   2 Tbsp. salsa
> 2 pieces whole wheat toast topped with
>   2 oz. herbed yogurt cheese*
> 1 orange

L: Quick & Easy Bagel
>   1 whole wheat bagel, halved and toasted, topped with:
>   2 Tbsp. natural peanut butter
>   1 banana, sliced
>   1 cup nonfat milk

Sn: Trail Mix
>   1/2 cup Wheat Chex® cereal
>   1/4 cup assorted dry fruit
>   2 Tbsp. nuts/seeds of choice
>   8 oz. nonfat light yogurt

> **People who need less than 2,000 calories a day, especially women, should maintain a high milk, yogurt, and cheese intake to provide necessary calcium.**

D: Salmon
>   3 oz. salmon fillet
>   marinate in 1/4 cup soy sauce, fresh ginger & garlic to
>   taste, then bake
>   1/2 cup steamed asparagus tips
>   topped with 1 tsp. butter
>   1/2 yam, sliced and oven grilled
>   topped with 1 tsp. butter
>   2/3 cup nonfat, sugar free ice cream topped with:
>   1/4 cup fresh berries
>   2 Tbsp. chopped nuts of choice

Nutrition Information: Day 3
Total Cal: 2078; % Carb: 53, % Fat: 27, % Pro: 20, SFAs+TFAs: 7%;
     Total Fiber: 45 g; Total Sugars: 100 g (≤ 10% is refined).

*Note: Yogurt cheese can easily be made by straining plain yogurt overnight in the refrigerator through either a very fine mesh strainer or cheesecloth. Discard the liquid portion and season the cheese as desired (i.e.: sun-dried tomatoes, onion and dill, roasted garlic and thyme - - be imaginative).

DAY 4

B: Breakfast Sandwich
>1 whole wheat English muffin, toasted
>1 whole egg, fried with non-stick spray
>2 pieces turkey bacon
>1/2 oz. reduced fat cheese

1 orange
1 cup nonfat milk

L: Quick Three Bean Chili
>1 Lean Cuisine Three Bean Chili® entree
>1/2 oz. reduced fat cheese
>2 tsp. light sour cream
>1 piece jalapeño corn bread, from mix
> topped with 1 tsp butter

1 cup watermelon
1 cup nonfat milk

> **The *Better Life Diet* provides
> healthy food with great taste
> for a long life.**

Sn: Filled Tortilla
>1/4 cup cooked black beans
>1/8 cup cooked brown rice
>1 oz. reduced fat cheese
>2 Tbsp. salsa
>1 whole wheat tortilla filled, folded, and fried in 1 tsp olive oil
>2 tsp. light sour cream

D: Pork Kabob
>marinade: 1/2 cup apple juice, 1 Tbsp olive oil, cloves, garlic, herbs
>marinate the following, then skewer with 2 bamboo spears & grill:
>>2 oz. pork tenderloin, cubed
>>1/2 cup potato, cubed
>>1/2 cup asparagus tips
>>1/2 apple, cubed
>>4 pearl onions

1/2 cup cooked brown & wild rice
1 cup nonfat milk
1 Dole® fruit juice bar

Nutrition Information: Day 4
Total Cal: 2010; % Carb: 50, % Fat: 28, % Pro: 22, SFAs+TFAs: 10%;
    Total Fiber: 35 g; Total Sugars: 91 g (≤ 10% is refined).

DAY 5

B: Oatmeal

      1 cup cooked oatmeal stir in:

            2 Tbsp. natural peanut butter

            1 packet Equal® sweetener

1 apple

1 cup nonfat milk

L: Turkey Sandwich

      2 pieces rye bread

      1 oz. skinless turkey breast

      top with:

> The *Better Life Diet* provides delicious food at low cost.

            1/2 oz. reduced fat cheese

            1/4 of an avocado

            1 tsp. Dijon mustard

            spinach, tomato, red onion, black olives to taste

2 kiwi

1 cup nonfat milk

Sn: English Muffin Pizza

      1 whole wheat English muffin, toasted

      top each half with:

            2 Tbsp. spaghetti sauce

            1/2 vegetarian sausage link, sliced

            1/4 oz. reduced fat cheese

D: Peanut Chicken Stir Fry

      3 oz. skinless chicken breast

      1 cup stir fried vegetables (snap peas, bell pepper, zucchini, carrots, broccoli, mushrooms)

      1 cup brown rice

      peanut sauce - heat in saucepan then pour over stir fry dish:

            2 Tbsp. each: Teriyaki sauce, natural peanut butter

            1/4 tsp. each: fresh chopped ginger, crushed red pepper chili flakes

            1 tsp. sesame oil

1 fortune cookie

1 cup Lipton® spiced chai tea, made with equal parts nonfat milk and water

1 packet Equal® sweetener

Nutrition Information: Day 5
Total Cal: 2038; % Carb: 50, % Fat: 29, % Pro: 21, SFAs+TFAs: 6.1%;
      Total Fiber: 45 g; Total Sugars: 88.6 g (≤ 10% is refined).

DAY 6

B: Breakfast Shake & Bagel
> 1/2 banana, frozen
> 1/2 cup each: frozen strawberries, orange juice, lowfat buttermilk
> 1/2 tsp. each: vanilla extract, nutmeg
> 1/2 whole wheat bagel
> 1 Tbsp. almond butter

L: Pita Sandwich & Soup
> 1/2 wheat pita pocket stuffed with:
>> 2 oz. skinless chicken breast
>> fresh spinach & artichoke hearts
>> 1 oz. feta cheese
>> red pepper pureé, blend together and spread inside pita:
>>> 2 oz. water packed roasted red pepper
>>> 2 tsp. olive oil
>>> 1 tsp. each: fresh parsley, capers, minced garlic
> 1 Nile Spice® Instant Minestrone cup of soup
> 1 orange
> 1 cup nonfat milk

Sn: Tuna & Crackers
> 1/4 cup water-packed tuna mixed with:
>> 2 Tbsp. chopped celery
>> 2 tsp. mayonnaise
> 8 Triscuits®
> 1 apple

Crash diets aren't the answer. The *Better Life Diet and Exercise Program* is the answer (pp. 150-152).

D: Spaghetti With Meat Sauce
> 1 cup vegetable sauce with:
>> 1/2 cup tomatoes
>> 1/4 cup each: zucchini, mushrooms
>> Italian spices to taste
>> 1 tsp. olive oil
> 2 oz. extra lean ground beef
> 1 1/2 cup whole wheat spaghetti noodles
> top pasta dish with
>> 1 Tbsp. each: pine nuts, parmesan cheese
> 1/2 baked pear

Nutrition Information: Day 6
Total Cal: 2012; % Carb: 53, % Fat: 28, % Pro: 19, SFAs+TFAs: 7.4%;
    Total Fiber: 42 g; Total Sugars: 98 g ($\leq$ 10 % is refined).

DAY 7 (fast food)

B: McDonald's
>1/2 Apple Bran Muffin
>1 serving pork sausage
>1 carton orange juice
>1 carton milk, 1 % *

L: Wendy's
>Grilled Chicken Sandwich
>Deluxe Garden Salad, nonfat dressing
>1 apple**
>1 carton milk, 2 % *

Sn: Muffin & Yogurt
>1/2 Apple Bran Muffin (from breakfast)
>8 oz. nonfat light yogurt**
>1 small box raisins**
>1/2 cup baby carrots**

D: Pizza Hut
>2 pieces Veggie Lover's® pizza
>1 orange**

> **Combine the *Better Life Diet* with two miles of continuous brisk walking daily and five minutes of lifting 3 to 6 lb. handweights slowly each morning and evening (pp. 166, 167, 174, 175).**

Nutrition Information: Day 7
Total Cal: 1894; % Carb: 51, % Fat: 30, % Pro: 19, SFAs+TFAs: 10%;
Total Fiber: 20.3 g; Total sugars: 128 g (≤ 10% is refined).

* Nonfat milk would be best. The milk designated, however, is the type that was sold at these fast food restaurants in the Seattle area at the time we wrote these sample meal plans.

** Indicates items that must be brought from home.

Note: This menu was included as an example of how to enjoy a balanced meal on the occasions that you eat at a fast food restaurant. As you can see, you do not need to totally eliminate these foods from your diet. Most fast foods, however, tend to have excess amounts of low-fiber carbohydrates, refined sugar, saturated fats, *trans* fatty acids, calories, and sodium. In addition, your body often does not get enough fresh fruits and vegetables when you eat out frequently.

Exercise -- *Essential Ally of Diet*

A diet without exercise is like a car with four flat tires. It can't go very far. This is why we emphasize that *exercise is the essential ally of diet.* But, exercise must be **aerobic** ("with oxygen") to benefit most of us. Aerobic exercise *doesn't* deplete your muscles of oxygen, make you short of breath, or cause you to perspire heavily (unless it's very warm). On the other hand, **anaerobic** ("without oxygen") exercise *does* deplete your muscles of oxygen, make you breathless and unable to speak, and cause you to perspire heavily.

Anaerobic exercise demands more oxygen and nutrients than your arterial blood can deliver to your overworked muscles. It also produces more waste products than your blood can remove. Such excessive exercise makes you severely short of breath, causes your pulse to race, and wears you out quickly. It's neither safe nor good for the average non-athletic person.

Aerobic exercise, however, is performed at a pace which is within the capacity of your circulation to deliver the extra oxygen and nutrients that your working muscles need. Your blood also removes the waste products from your muscles that activity produces. You can continue this rhythmic muscular activity for long periods with a stable, moderately elevated pulse rate without becoming breathless, exhausted, or drenched in sweat. Aerobic exercise is safe and good for you. Combine it with the **Better Life Diet** for health and happiness.

The ability to talk while exercising *(the talk test)* is a simple way to tell whether an exercise is "aerobic" for you. If you can carry on a normal conversation, it is; if you can't, it's anaerobic. People in poor shape fail the *test* while walking slowly; people in good shape pass while walking briskly; people in excellent shape pass while jogging. Regardless of the activity, adjust your pace so you can pass the "*test*."

Regular aerobic exercise:

- **Costs little in time or money.**
- **Uses calories.**
- **Increases joy in life.**
- **Tones and enlarges muscles.**
- **Sharpens your mind.**
- **Alleviates depression.**
- **Reduces stress.**

- **Promotes sound sleep.**
- **Strengthens heart and lungs.**
- **Lowers risk of osteoporosis.**
- **Assists the whole body to use oxygen and nutrients more efficiently.**
- **Helps the digestive system to work better.**
- **Improves dangerous blood chemistries.**

Walking is of special value to women after menopause because the cyclic impacting effect of weight bearing with each alternating step acts to slow the development of osteoporosis, a process that absorbs bone structure and weakens the skeleton. This effect is enhanced by the *Better Life Diet* and by taking vitamin D, calcium, magnesium, and estrogens or related non-hormonal compounds (p. 88).

Severe osteoporosis weakens bones so much, especially of the hips, spine, ribs, and wrists that they break easily. This occurs more often in elderly women than men, at a ratio of about 4:1. Even without obvious fractures of the backbone, osteoporosis silently shortens the spine of both men and women and causes them to lose height in their advancing years. Walking tends to stop this "melting away" of bone.

A few points need emphasis. We all need aerobic exercise to help strengthen bones, increase muscle size and power, lose excess stored fat (weight), improve heart and lung function, and gain a renewed sense of vigor. These benefits of aerobic exercise promote fitness and help prevent osteoporosis, obesity, type 2 diabetes (p. 279), blindness, kidney failure, hypertension, atherosclerosis, clots, heart attacks, sudden cardiac death, congestive heart failure, strokes, decreased exercise capacity, limb loss, and aneurysm formation. In brief, regular aerobic exercise is the closest thing we have to an **"anti-aging pill."** You'll find that life's a lot more fun when you take this "pill" every day.

Walking briskly without becoming winded is hard to beat as an exercise for many reasons. It's safe, pleasant, inexpensive, good for most everything, and able to be enjoyed nearly any time and any place. Try it! Two miles in the morning or evening will do wonders for you. This is a habit to form, combine with **The Better Life Diet,** and practice for life.

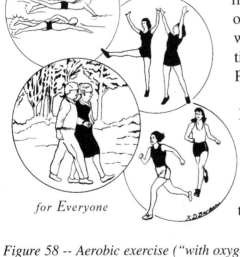

There is an Aerobic Exercise

for Everyone

Walk with your husband, wife, children, friend, or dog. If none of them are available, walk alone. This is time you owe yourself. Precious time.

If you can't walk two miles, try one. If not one, do what is comfortable for you and slowly increase the distance.

Figure 58 -- Aerobic exercise ("with oxygen") is good "every day medicine." But if you are seriously overweight, and/or have heart trouble, or other illness, please contact your physician for guidance before beginning an exercise program.

F.I.T.
The Basics:
F̲requency ... I̲ntensity ... T̲ime

The first thing to know about "regular aerobic exercise" is that unless you do it *frequently enough, intensely enough,* and *long enough,* it's not going to do you, your cardiovascular, respiratory, or muscular systems, or your weight reduction program much good.

As an aid to getting in shape and staying that way, think F.I.T. for the **frequency**, **intensity**, and **time** of exercise.

Frequency

The American College of Sports Medicine recommends daily aerobic exercise to achieve fitness. I agree and believe that we need daily exercise just as much as we need to eat everyday. We need to use our muscles consistently to keep them and our heart and lungs in shape. There's no way around this requirement. *We either use our muscles or we lose them* -- an easy choice if we wish to get in shape and stay fit.

Intensity

Most of the mystique that surrounds aerobic exercise has to do with its intensity or "pace."

Take *"the talk test"* to find the aerobic pace that's right for you (pp. 161, 162). Increase your pace to where you can't carry a conversation and then slow down to where you can. Don't exercise on the "edge." You need some "breathing room."

When you're in the "groove," you'll work up a moderate

sweat, but you won't get breathless. If you find yourself huffing and puffing and unable to carry on a conversation, slow down and find the pace that's right for you. Leave long distance running and triathlon competition to the athletes. It's not healthy for you to go to the edge of your endurance. *A daily, brisk 2-mile walk and lifting 3 lb. handweights slowly for 5 minutes each A.M. and P.M. are superb exercises* (p. 167). You will find them easy to perform, enjoyable, and effective.

Time

Many studies show that we need at least 30 minutes of aerobic exercise most days of the week for reasonable fitness.

There is some controversy here, however. A panel of experts convened by the American College of Sports Medicine and the Centers for Disease Control (CDC) recently announced that *accumulating* 30 minutes of "moderate exercise" each day (e.g., walking, gardening, climbing several flights of stairs, and/or doing housework *every* day) is enough to improve overall fitness, at least moderately. Researchers at the Harvard School of Public Health believe, instead, that 45 minutes of daily, brisk, *continuous* exercise is preferable.

The bottom line is that even a *little* exercise is better than no exercise, and in general, *more* exercise is better than less exercise -- within reason of course.

Thirty minutes of daily aerobic exercise will help you attain and maintain your optimal weight. If you need to lose weight faster, perform 45 to 60 minutes of continuous aerobic exercise once or, if necessary, twice a day. This need not be complicated. Just go out, start walking, and build from there.

Questions and Answers About Exercise

Q. *What are the different types of exercise?*

A. 1. *Isometric exercise* (muscle contraction without motion) tones the tensed muscles, but uses few calories.This type of exercise doesn't improve *overall* cardiovascular, respiratory, or muscular fitness.

2. *Isotonic exercise* (muscle contraction with motion, *e.g.,* weight lifting) is far more valuable than isometric exercise. Lifting heavy weights, however, is not practical for most middle-aged and older people. *But doing several sets of lifting 3 to 6 lb. handweights slowly to the point of some muscle fatigue daily is practical.* This simple routine builds arm, shoulder, back, and pectoral muscle size and strength. Increased muscle mass raises your metabolic rate which burns more stored fat even while you're resting (p. 185).

3. *Anaerobic exercise (without* adequate oxygen) -- such as sprinting or fast cycling -- quickly leads to exhaustion and breathlessness. Physical benefits are difficult to realize when the body is running short of oxygen. Also, severe anaerobic exercise can be dangerous for the non-trained person because it quickly depletes the heart of oxygen.

4. *Aerobic exercises (with* adequate oxygen) such as **walking**, dancing, jogging, golfing (preferably without a cart), cycling, swimming, handball, tennis, and rowing can be continued for long periods without becoming breathless if your pace is right. These exercises build muscle, get your heart and

lungs in shape, help you attain and maintain a healthful weight, and keep you in good condition. **This combination of benefits could save your life!**

Q. *Should I check with my doctor before beginning an exercise program?*

A. Yes, if you:
- Are 35 years of age, or older.
- Haven't seen your physician for over a year.
- Have a personal or family history of cardiovascular disease.
- Are a smoker, or have high blood pressure.
- Are seriously overweight.

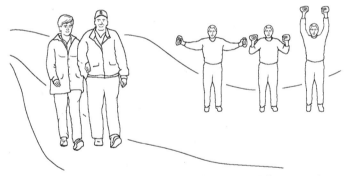

Special Note: It is important to find aerobic exercises that you *like* to do. There are many for you to choose from in this section. My favorites are those shown above. At age 74, I greatly enjoy briskly walking two miles each evening with my wife. Also, I enjoy lifting three-pound weights in a slow, repetitive, stretching (reach the sky or horizon) manner for five minutes each morning and evening. I am confident that this practical exercise routine, requiring about 45 minutes a day, could also help you enjoy a long and youthful life. *Be innovative in developing an effective, **daily** program that you like. There is much to choose from (pp. 161-187).*

Q. *How can I find time to exercise?*

A. The same way you find time every day to eat and sleep. Exercise is just as important. **Make it a real priority because exercise is vital!**

Q. *What are my exercise choices?*

A. There are many. The following comments about the more popular aerobic exercises are to pique your interest and get you involved.

1. Aerobics

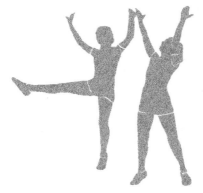

Special Advantages:

- Special fun for those who like exercising to music. Such music can sway your soul.
- Entire body is exercised.
- Group spirit is established in the classes.
- Necessary skill is rapidly acquired. Beginners become "pros" in a short time.
- Classes are held inside, away from the weather.
- Many styles of aerobics and different kinds of music to choose from.

Special Equipment, Facilities, and Personnel Needed:

- Loose-fitting clothing and comfortable shoes with cushioned soles (athletic shoes give the best support).
- Space and a qualified instructor.

Advice for Beginners:

- Talk to your friends and find out what program and which instructor they enjoy and why. If that doesn't work, check with the registered programs in your community, such as those at the YWCA or YMCA, and ask what they offer. Then talk to their instructors.

- Sign up for classes with a friend. You'll encourage each other and have lots of fun.

- The typical aerobic dance program consists of a one-hour class Monday, Wednesday, and Friday for three months. But some aerobics classes are only offered twice a week. Unfortunately, such schedules don't provide enough exercise to get your cardiovascular, respiratory, and muscular systems in good shape. To get more exercise, sign up for an additional program, or supplement your classes with other aerobic exercises that you do on your own, such as walking or swimming.

- Make sure you exercise strenuously enough in your class to work up a moderate sweat, but don't get so carried away that you become breathless and drenched in sweat.

2. Cycling

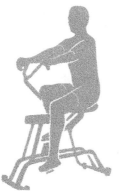

Special Advantages:

- Especially well-suited for older and overweight individuals, and for those with back, knee, and/or foot problems.

- Outdoor bikes can be used for transportation.

- Indoor bikes protect you from the weather and allow you to watch television while pedaling.

Special Equipment Needed:

- An outdoor or indoor bike. These may be purchased or rented from a cycle shop. Want ads and garage sales may be useful in finding a good second-hand bike.

- Before purchasing a bike, check consumer magazines, read a bicycle book, and talk with friends. If you still need more guidance, consult a fitness professional. Then comparison shop.

- Outdoor bikes should have at least three gears.

- Indoor bikes *must* have an adjustable tension control. All other special features are optional.

Advice for Beginners:

- Have a bike specialist "fit" your bike to your body by adjusting the seat and handle bar heights and positions so your legs and back are comfortable

- Outdoor cyclists should wear helmets because they provide needed protection against devastating head (brain) injuries in case of an accident.

- Work on finding a pedaling pace and tension control that will give you an adequate workout without causing shortness of breath. If you get to the point of breathlessness, slow down until you catch your breath. Then pick your pace up to the point you're sweating some but aren't winded. Continue at this speed.

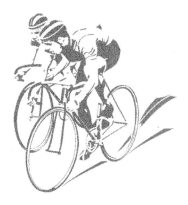

3. Swimming

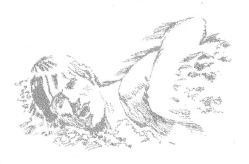

Special Advantages:

- Well-suited for most everyone who can swim and especially those with back and/or joint problems which restrict or prohibit them from enjoying other popular aerobic exercises.

- The perfect aerobic exercise for those who want a good workout but hate to sweat.

- Works on all body muscles.

Special Equipment and Facilities Needed:

- Swim suit.

- Eye and ear protection, if necessary.

- A swimming pool. Check out the pools operated by the parks department, YMCA, YWCA, and local health clubs. Be sure that the pool you select is large enough for nonstop lap swimming. You need space for this.

Advice for Beginners:

- Inquire when your pool opens and closes. Some run from 5:00 A.M. to 10:00 P.M. Avoid the crowded times. Even fish need room to swim.

- Use any stroke and get in as much nonstop lane swimming as possible during your exercise time. If you start to lose your breath, slow down. Once you've caught your breath, find your proper stroke and pace.

- If it's difficult for you to get to a pool on a regular basis, use the other suggested aerobic exercises to supplement your swimming program. In doing this, don't forget how important it is that you enjoy your daily exercise routine. Make it fun!

Swimming and Osteoporosis:

- Studies have shown that swimming *doesn't* strengthen your bones. If you're concerned about osteoporosis, get plenty of *weight-bearing* exercise, *such as walking*, which does strengthen your bones (p. 162).

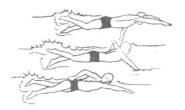

4. Walking

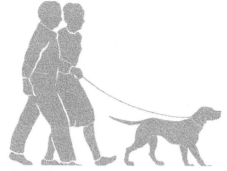

Special Advantages:

- This is the best exercise for the great majority of us because it's easily within our capabilities, is an enjoyable challenge to our bodies, and is a rich source of health benefits (pp. 162, 163).

- Two miles of brisk walking daily increases *nitric oxide* production (p. 176) and is superb exercise for the young and not-so-young, alike.

- Excellent for short-distance transportation.

- Provides the same benefits as jogging but with less risk of injury.

- No expertise is needed; you've been doing it since you were one year old.

Special Equipment Needed:

- Comfortable shoes with cushioned soles that give you good, stable support - - that's all you need. You can't beat this for simplicity.

Advice for Beginners:

- If you're out of shape, begin slowly and first increase the distance and then your pace, but do this in a careful, progressive manner. If you become breathless or don't feel comfortable, you're going too fast -- slow down! When you've caught your breath, continue at the upper pace that still enables you to talk normally.

- Over a period of weeks to months, work up to a level where you can briskly walk nonstop for 30 to 60 minutes without feeling winded.

- Don't count the stop-and-go, casual walking you do around the house or at the office as part of your walking program. Stop-and-go exercises don't provide enough conditioning benefits for your heart and lungs. Set special time aside for brisk, nonstop walking. These are precious moments *you owe yourself.*

- Overweight people find that the addition of nonstop, brisk walking to their daily routines can help them lose weight without having to severely reduce their caloric intake.

- When you reach a point where you need more of a challenge, strap on a weighted backpack or add a few hills to your walking program.

- Notes on brisk-walking form: swing your arms, take long strides, and look at the beautiful world around you. *Remember that you are an important part of this scene, too.*

5. Jogging

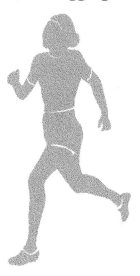

Special Advantages:

- Jogging is effective in increasing the production of *nitric oxide* by the endothelial cells that line our blood vessels. This causes the small arteries to enlarge and the blood flow to increase. Nitric oxide also makes the vessel lining smooth and slippery. These changes reduce clot and plaque formation.

- It's fun and motivating to jog with a companion if you like company during exercise. Pick a buddy, however, who's approximately at your level of fitness. If he or she is in much better shape, you will be run ragged. But, if your companion lags far behind in speed and/or stamina, you'll find it hard to get to the level of exercise that you need.

Special Equipment Needed:

- Quality running shoes (not sneakers) are essential to protect your feet and joints from the pounding they take in jogging. Shoes should extend 3/4" beyond the longest toe, fit perfectly over athletic socks, allow no slippage of the heel, be sufficiently flexible (even when new) to be comfortable, and have shock-absorbing soles.

- Hundreds of brands and varieties of running shoes are available. Shop around until you find a perfect fit. In general, athletic stores tend to have wider selections and more experienced salespeople.

- Dress in layers when it's cold; don't overdress when it's warm.

- If you have knee and/or foot problems, you may need to see an orthopedist or a podiatrist to obtain special instructions and/or an orthotic shoe insert.

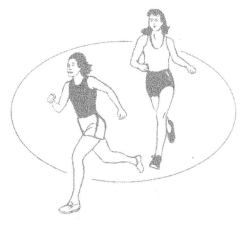

Beginning Jogging

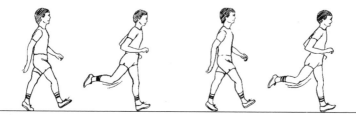

Alternate walking with slow jogging.

Advice for Beginners:

- Invest in a good book on jogging before beginning your program.

- At first, alternate walking with slow jogging, slowing to a walk whenever you reach the point where you can't talk normally. Gradually increase the proportion of jogging time to walking time until you are jogging on a nonstop basis. Don't expect too much too soon. You will get there. Be patient!

- If you feel you are able to do more, extend your time, not your speed (pace).

- Don't try to keep up with others who are in better shape than you. Exercise at your own pace. *You* are in charge!

- Take time to "warm up" and stretch. This is important to help prevent injuries.
- Stay within your improving exercise capacity.
- Don't lean forward when you jog.
- Hold your forearms approximately parallel to the ground, and keep your hands and shoulders relaxed.
- Keep your stride short -- don't let your feet get out ahead of your knees.
- Land on your heels, not on the balls of your feet. Sore feet are no fun.
- Breathe through your mouth.
- When you're within about 10 minutes of stopping your exercise session, slow your jogging pace down gradually *and finish by walking at a comfortable pace for several more minutes.* This allows time for your circulation to clear the lactic acid from your muscles in order to avoid having them become stiff and sore. Treat your muscles with respect.

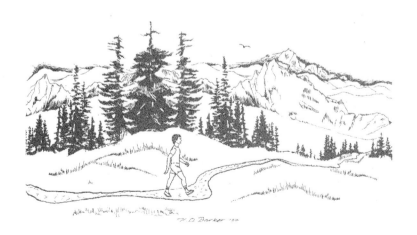

Times to Exercise

Before Breakfast

Advantages:

- Raises your metabolic rate early in the day.
- Clears your mind and invigorates your body so you can begin your day with enthusiasm.
- At this refreshing time of day, it's hard to make excuses for not exercising.
- You have to take a shower anyway.

Possible Disadvantages:

- It may be hard to get out of bed a little earlier.

Before Lunch

Advantages:

- Works off morning tensions.
- Refreshes you to meet the afternoon demands.
- Helps curb lunch appetite.

Possible Disadvantages:

- You may need to shower and not have an opportunity to do so.
- Your lunch break may not be long enough for you to complete an adequate exercise session and still have time to eat.

Before Dinner

Advantages:

- Clears away the day's worries.
- Refreshes you for evening activities.
- Helps curb dinner appetite.

Possible Disadvantages:

- Easy to find a reason not to exercise at this time of day.

After Dinner

Advantages:

- Clears your mind and helps you relax.
- Walking following eating helps your digestive system to work better and doesn't require waiting. (Both my wife and I like to take our evening walk shortly after we have cleared the dinner table and put the dishes in the dishwasher.)

Possible Disadvantages:

- Easy to say -- "It's late, I'll do it tomorrow."
- You may need to wait for an hour or more after you have eaten before doing certain types of exercise, such as jogging or calisthenics.

There are a million excuses for not exercising regularly. Here are a few:

"I don't have the time."

All it takes is a minimum of 30 minutes of aerobic exercise most days to stay in reasonable shape. You'll be set if you take 10 minutes from your usual TV watching time, 10 minutes from your sleep time, and 10 minutes from your goof-off time and use these minutes for vital aerobic exercise everyday. You can't lose with this trade-off - - a real bargain!

"I don't have the energy."

The vast majority of people who exercise regularly say exercise makes them "feel full of energy," and that's why they do it. Exercise, by getting the blood circulating and the muscles moving, is an ideal way to overcome frustration, relieve stress, and clear your mind of the day's problems. In this way, it serves to supply you with more energy, providing a kind of "second wind" that recharges your batteries.

"I always get sore."

Sore muscles result from doing too much, too soon, and not coming to a gradual stop. Start a routine where you gradually increase the time of exercising before increasing the speed (pace). Before stopping, slow down gradually over 5 to 10 minutes, so your muscles won't become stiff and sore (p. 179).

"It's too much work to get in shape."

A nice thing about aerobic exercise is that you can adjust the pace to suit your needs. You'll soon find the right speed that will allow you to progressively extend your exercise time to 30 minutes without becoming breathless.

"I've tried getting more exercise, but I never stick with it."

This time you will! You can afford 30 minutes of aerobic exercise on most days of the week. No big deal! If you need a motivator, exercise with a buddy, use gold stars on a calendar, or anything that works for you. The key is to *make exercise a high priority* and develop it into a faithful habit.

"I'm too old."

You're only as old as you feel and regular exercise makes you feel younger. Start slowly, and work on *gradually* increasing your muscular, cardiovascular, and respiratory endurances.

"I hate fighting the weather."

An indoor swimming pool, exercycle, shopping mall (for walking), or an aerobics class can help. If these don't suit your fancy, get a treadmill, and walk *inside* on rainy days.

"I have arthritis."

Your doctor may recommend that you cycle or swim indoors, or do both. Studies show that these exercises will help relieve your arthritic pains and stiffness and limber you up.

"I'm too busy running around doing things for other people."

In order to help others more effectively, you must first take care of yourself. A half-hour of aerobic exercise most days is a gift you *must* give yourself. It will allow you to feel and look your best, and enable you to do more for others.

"Exercise is boring!"

Well, see what you can do to make it fun! Vary your walking/jogging route. Listen to music. Position your indoor bike so you can watch the evening news while you pump away. Join an aerobic dance class. Exercise with a friend. Treat yourself to new athletic shoes. Challenge yourself.

"I don't know what to do with the kids."

Don't worry. There are many possiblilities depending on your children's ages. If older, they could come with you. They need exercise, too! You could get a walking/jogging stroller for small children and take your son or daughter for a ride. If you use a health club, check whether they have child day-care. You may also wish to get a treadmill or an indoor bicycle and exercise at home -- with the kids!

"My family isn't interested."

That's okay. This is something you're doing for yourself.

"I'm not that interested in fitness; I've got other priorities."

Stop for a moment and reflect: "Exercise will help me live longer and better." And that's for real! And there's more.

Difficult problems often "solve themselves" while you exercise. This isn't an illusion. Exercise refreshes your mind and helps you think more clearly.

"I don't have the right clothes, equipment, etc."

Buy them. It could be one of the most valuable investments of your life. Why not? You owe this to yourself.

"I'm too fat."

So -- you're just the one who needs to exercise. Start with something easy, like walking around the block. Do that for a week. Go around twice the next week, and so on. See how much better you'll feel -- and how much less you'll want to eat! Keep at it, and you'll begin to feel better and better as you progressively lose excess fat while you gain needed muscle. Don't forget that losing excess fat stores is just a matter of using more calories than you take in.

"According to the charts, I'd have to jog forever just to work off one doughnut."

Exercise charts only tell half the story. *First* of all, many people find that regular aerobic exercise is a powerful appetite suppressant because it reduces tension and depression, common causes of the "munchies." Exercise also signals the hormone, glucagon, to convert some of the liver's glycogen into glucose and release it into the blood, which helps to further curb the appetite.

Second, muscles that are exercised on a regular basis use more energy (calories) even when resting than muscles which have not been exercised. Exercise "tunes" the body's engines (muscles) so they idle faster at rest.

In addition, the muscles of people who exercise on a regular basis get bigger. As a consequence, fit people, pound per pound, burn more calories than fat people because a pound of resting muscle burns more calories than a pound of fat. This difference in caloric consumption becomes even more

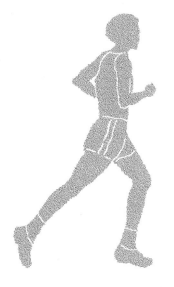

pronounced after exercising and lasts for many hours.

Have faith. If you have a large amount of fat to lose and are only losing one pound per week, don't get discouraged. You're on track. Fifty pounds in a year is a lot. Remember, the right way to lose weight permanently is to lose excess stored fat gradually while you add muscle (pp. 150-152).

"I will just exercise the fat parts of my body."

It's true that fat tends to accumulate in specific areas of the body. It generally shows up around the waists of men (apple shape) and the hips and thighs of women (pear shape).

Spot-reduction exercises like sit-ups and leg-lifts make the abdominal muscles stronger and firmer. The same fat deposits, however, still sit on top of those muscles. The fat on top of a muscle does not belong to that muscle; it belongs to the whole body. This fat will begin to "melt away" only when the demand for calories in the whole body exceeds the caloric intake. We keep coming back to this basic fact.

In general, spot-reduction exercises don't use as much energy as whole-body aerobic exercises, such as walking or jogging. These whole-body exercises are better because they use larger sets of muscles and require more calories to meet the increased energy requirements. And when you use more calories than you eat, you lose weight. Simple as that.

Remember, excess stored fat depresses the metabolic rate, while added muscle increases it. The more muscle you have, the more fat you will burn. You must also reduce your blood insulin level by severely restricting **low-fiber** carbohydrates and refined sugar (pp. 138, 144, 152). This dietary strategy enables your stored fat to be used for energy.

Special Note: I advise plastic surgery for removal of fat deposits *only* when these deposits are very persistent and disfiguring. A currently popular operation for this purpose is called **liposuction**. In this procedure, the plastic surgeon inserts a tubular suction device through the skin and uses it to slim and contour the excessively padded areas by literally sucking out the adipose tissue. Though this technique is indicated for some patients, it's an **expensive and potentially dangerous way to lose fat.** In most cases, there is a better way: *The Better Life Diet and Exercise Program!*

"I had coronary bypass surgery three weeks ago, and I don't know if it's safe for me to begin an exercise program."

If you are gaining strength, feeling better, and able to walk up a flight or two of stairs without becoming short of breath or developing chest pain, your doctor will be delighted! In fact, he or she will likely start you on a progressive walking program at that point.

Your physician will follow your progress closely. When you are ready, he or she will extend the distance you walk and, later, increase your pace. Your doctor may also refer you to a cardiac rehabilitation program near your home. There are good programs in most areas of the United States today. They promote proper diet, exercise, health education, and confidence.

Exercise is an important part of both your short-term and long-term treatment plans. Don't become impatient and go too fast early on, or become too busy to exercise later on.

Remember, the time you take to exercise is a precious gift you owe yourself and your loved ones. *Make your combined diet and exercise program a high priority* because it is vital for you to enjoy a long and youthful life in the years ahead.

<u>Stress</u> -- *Potential Killer*

Stress is the summation of all our emotional, mental, and physical responses to the threatening inner and outer conflicts that challenge us everyday. While some stress helps us stay sharp and responsive, too much stress is destructive. This turbulent state causes us to become tense, irritable, apprehensive, and frightened. Stress causes the adrenal glands to make and release a flood of adrenalin which makes our pulse race, small arteries constrict, blood pressure climb, heart work harder, and platelets become stickier. These changes can cause a heart attack. To stay out of this danger zone may require that we gain a greater understanding of ourselves, change our attitudes and goals, and obtain better control of our responses to the seemingly adverse situations that appear to surround and confront us. But how to do this?

Difficulty in maintaining a suitable balance between our past, present, and future in this incredible age of discovery, change, and turmoil can become a source of unbearable tension for any of us.

We need **balance** in our lives because otherwise we may live too much in the future or too much in the past. Although we must learn from the past to plan for the future and be inspired by what is yet to come, our focal point should be the ever present now because that's the reality of life.

The best defense against developing excessive stress in response to the many challenges in our lives is to maintain a happy, relaxed mental state by doing God's work in the here and now to the full extent of our abilities and leaving the rest to Him. We can do this best by helping those who need us in a spirit of love. When we do this, God rewards us with a joyful life that is free of anxiety, fear, and worry.

Being kind, thoughtful, and generous to others is the surest way for any of us to find peace and happiness in each day of our lives. Since we all yearn for this mental state, why not go for it by following this "can't miss" agenda?

This plan for peace of mind, serenity of soul, and exhilaration of spirit could be more effective than the billions of dollars spent yearly in the United States on tranquilizers, mood elevators, and sedatives to combat fear, loneliness, and simple depression. And not only would we be happier people, our homes, cities, states, nation, and world would also be better.

Our time on earth passes all too quickly. In fact, our earthly lives will be over almost before we realize what has happened to us. All find this inevitable reality difficult to comprehend. We need help to accept and fully appreciate the beauty of what this reality can be.

The late, beloved Mother Teresa tells us how to defuse our anxiety in the Foreword she wrote for the book, ***The Open Heart***. In that message, she affirms that the way to peace and joy in our personaly journeys to eternity is to serve those in need with love and joy in our hearts.

There is infinite wisdom in the *universal prayer of St. Francis* (p. 270). You may wish to memorize it. The simple repetition of this prayer each day will bring greater peace and joy to all who do so. I say this prayer each morning and evening. In the morning, St. Francis's words bring focus to what my day could be and at night to what it has been. This reflection reduces the stress in my life. I believe that it could do the same for you, too.

Section IV:

A Simple Nonsurgical Plan for a Long and Youthful Life

- General Considerations 191-192

- The Five Cardinal Rules for
  Heart-Healthy (Fit) Living 192-195

- Three Additional Strategies 196-199

  1. Take Antioxidants and
     Homocysteine-Lowering Vitamins 197

  2. Reduce the Stickiness of
     Your Platelets if They
     Are Too Sticky... 198

  3. Select a Good Doctor and
     Follow His or Her Advice................................ 199

Preventable fatalities (p. 191) account for about 75% of all premature deaths in the US. Adherence to the *Five Cardinal Rules for Heart-Healthy (Fit) Living* will help you avoid these fatal illnesses and extend your life.

General Considerations

Heart attack and stroke are the leading killers in the industrial world. But the good news is that the death rate for cardiovascular disease in the U.S. has decreased about 20% in recent years. But the rising incidence of obesity and type 2 diabetes threatens to reverse this favorable trend. There is still much for us to do.

Hardening of the arteries (atherosclerosis) begins early in life. *Autopsy examinations of adolescent American accident victims have shown extensive fatty plaques in the coronaries of many high-school students.* These findings indicate that we must start in childhood to prevent heart and other deadly diseases from developing. This can be done by teaching today's children the rules of heart-healthy (fit) living in three interrelated ways:

1. Good example and instruction by parents in the home. This is vital!
2. Positive guidance by pediatricians and family physicians.
3. Proper training by teachers in the schools.

"An ounce of *prevention* in early years is worth a pound of *cure* in later years." But preventive efforts must be both *simple* and *effective* if they are to be widely adopted as a way of life. Our rules pass this test. Simply said, they are: *don't smoke, closely follow the **Better Life Diet and Exercise Program**, attain and maintain a healthful weight, and control stress* (p. 193 and Fig. 59, p. 194). In brief, prevention in the key, not more surgery.

These rules will help you avoid obesity, type 2 diabetes (p. 279), blindness, kidney failure, atherosclerosis, hypertension, clots, heart attacks, sudden cardiac death, congestive heart failure, strokes, decreased walking capacity, limb loss, aneurysms, hemorrhages, many types of cancer (especially of the lung), emphysema, gallstones, and degenerative arthritis.

In addition, these guidelines are vital if you have had surgery
for heart or artery disease. This is because surgery is only a
mechanical solution to a structural problem caused by the
biochemical disorder, atherosclerosis (pp. 272, 273).

All arteries will eventually wear out if given enough time. In
earlier years so many people died of infections (such as
smallpox, pneumonia, influenza, typhoid, diphtheria,
tuberculosis, staph infections, strep infections, meningitis, and
appendicitis) that few lived long enough for this to happen. In
fact, most people died before reaching age 50. Now that we are
living longer (the average life span in the U.S. is about 74 years
for men and 79 for women), about *half* of us will die
prematurely from hardened arteries and clots unless we take
steps now to prevent this from happening later.

The Five Cardinal Rules
for
Heart-Healthy (Fit) Living

To increase our chances of living to a ripe old age with our
mental faculties and physical capabilities in top form, it's
necessary to follow an effective strategy to keep our arteries in
good condition. We have a multidimensional fitness plan to do
this and more. Our plan may be expressed through the
following five letters: **S ... D-E-W ... S** which identify the
targets of the five cardinal rules for heart-healthy (fit) living:

Smoking ... Diet-Exercise-Weight ... Stress

The plan works in two main ways: *First*, it protects the arterial
wall against atherosclerosis by lowering high blood levels of
LDL cholesterol, triglycerides, glucose, and homocysteine
while elevating low levels of HDL cholesterol and omega-3
fatty acids. *Second,* it decreases the ability of the blood to clot
by lowering high levels of fibrinogen and platelet stickiness.

The Rules

#1
Smoking

Don't smoke, or be around those who are smoking. This helps to prevent atherosclerosis, clots, heart attacks, strokes, limb loss, cancer (esp. lung), and emphysema. *Also, don't take other destructive drugs.*

#2
Diet

Follow the **Better Life Diet** (pp. 136-160), a meal plan consisting of high-fiber carbs, protective fats, and good proteins. This diet severely restricts low-fiber carbs, refined sugars, saturated fats, and *trans* fatty acids. It helps prevent obesity, type 2 diabetes (p. 279), hypertension, atherosclerosis, clots, heart attacks, sudden death, congestive failure, aneurysms, strokes, decreased walking capacity, limb loss, cancer, blindness, kidney failure, gallstones, and degenerative arthritis. This healthy diet is also delicious. The engaging taste of its many foods makes eating a joy to anticipate and a pleasure to realize (Fig. 60, p. 195).

#3
Exercise

Perform 45 minutes of **aerobic exercise** each day (pp. 161-187). Two miles of nonstop brisk walking daily and 5 minutes of repetitive lifting 3 to 6 lb. handweights in a slow, stretching (reach the sky or horizon) manner each morning and evening are excellent means to improve your fitness (p. 167).

#4
Weight

Attain and maintain your **ideal weight**. This is the weight at which you both feel and look your best.

#5
Stress

Strive for the **inner peace** that allows you to willingly accept problems as a challenging part of life. You can best achieve this mental state free of harmful stress by traveling the road of the ***Golden Rule*** to loving human relations.

The 5 Cardinal Rules for Heart-Healthy (Fit) Living

D
S . . . E . . . S
W

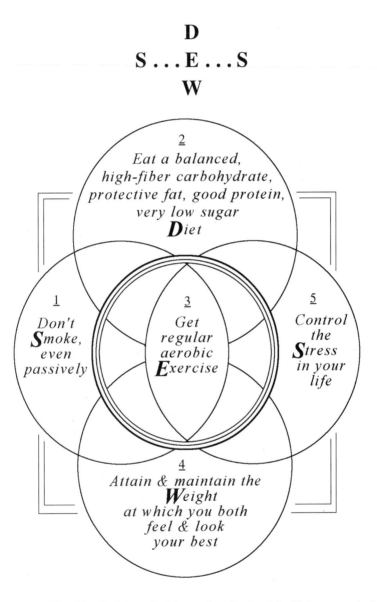

Figure 59 - The five interlocking rules for healthy living are vital for a long and youthful life (for diet, see p. 138 & Fig. 57, p.139).

Eat for Health and Taste
Protect Your Arteries
& Enjoy Life

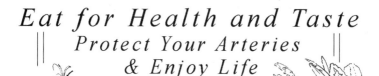

Fresh fruits,
fresh vegetables,
& legumes*

Fish &
poultry without skin

Eggs,** may have 1-2 per day

Drink nonfat milk

Whole grain breads, cereals,
& pastas*

Markedly restrict low-fiber carbohydrates
(white bread, mashed potatoes,
french fries, & white rice)

Drastically restrict refined sugar

Severely restrict saturated fat,
and <u>trans</u> fatty acids

* High-fiber, low glycemic index (p. 284) foods

** For people who don't have either diabetes or
elevated LDL cholesterol and/or triglycerides
(For those who do, see pp. 146, 276, 279, and 281)

*Figure 60 -- **The Better Life Diet** --*
Delicious foods that are good for you.

__Three Additional Strategies__

If people would follow the 5 cardinal rules for heart-healthy (fit) living, the incidence of heart attacks, strokes, limb loss, cancer, hypertension, obesity, type 2 diabetes, blindness, and kidney failure would drop dramatically. But some need more. These are the people who have a family or personal history of heart or artery disease at a young age (35 - 40 years) or have one or more of the following threatening blood chemistries:

1. An HDL cholesterol level below 35 mg/dL in men and below 45 mg/dL in women. The higher this value the better because HDL transports LDL cholesterol out of the blood and the arterial wall.

2. A fasting blood glucose > 120 mg/dL or a hemoglobin A1c value > 7%. (Under 100 mg/dL or under 6% is best.)

3. A fasting triglyceride level above 200 mg/dL. A value of under 100 is ideal. (Triglycerides are fats derived both from the fatty foods in our diet and from the conversion of excess carbohydrates and proteins into glucose which is converted into saturated fat.)

4. An LDL cholesterol level above 130 mg/dL. The *ideal* value for this lipid is under 100 mg/dL.

5. A fibrinogen level above 350 mg/dL. (Fibrinogen forms clots -- a value of 200 - 250 mg/dL is ideal.)

6. An increased platelet stickiness (causes clots).

7. An elevated homocysteine level. (see next page).

These people need the following three *additional strategies:*

1. Take Antioxidants and Homocysteine-Lowering Vitamins

"Free radical" is a popular term used to explain nearly everything that goes wrong in the body from cancer to heart disease and from arthritis to cataracts. This term refers to atoms (mainly oxygen) that have lost electrons. These electron-deficient (oxidized) atoms, as in tobacco smoke (p. 120), damage neighboring atoms by taking their electrons.

Current theory suggests that only the oxidized form of low-density lipoprotein cholesterol (LDL) damages the arterial wall. If further studies show this to be true, determination of the blood level of oxidized LDL will be important in the prediction of an individual's risk of developing a heart attack.

Chemicals that prevent free radicals from doing damage are called "antioxidants." Of foods with such properties (as fruits, vegetables, legumes, nuts, and seeds), blueberries have the most. In addition to enjoying a healthy, nutritious diet, protect yourself further against these "radicals" by taking antioxidant vitamins (50 mg of vitamin B6, 500 mg of vitamin C, 400 units of vitamin E), and 200 mcg of the antioxidant mineral selenium daily (costing together about 25 cents/day). Also, we suggest that people with multiple risk factors, including those on "statin" drugs, take 30 mg of the powerful antioxidant coenzyme Q-10 daily. Furthermore, we suggest that you take 400 mcg of folic acid, and 500 mcg of vitamin B12, along with the previously mentioned 50 mg of B6 daily to reduce your blood level of *homocysteine*. High concentrations of this amino acid (above 12 micromols/L) injure endothelial cells and predispose the inner arterial wall to develop atherosclerosis. A value below 8 micromols is best. Risk factors for elevated homocysteine levels parallel those for atherosclerosis (pp. 272, 273).

2. Reduce the Stickiness of Your Platelets if They Are Too Sticky

The degree of stickiness that platelets can develop is unique to each person. Platelets that become *very sticky* can cause fatal blood clots. Such platelets may *adhere, activate,* and *aggregate* on the diseased flow surface of atherosclerotic arteries, especially when soft plaques rupture and release their deadly lipid contents into the blood. These platelet aggregates may cause harmful clots to form which can block the channel and stop the flow of blood to vital regions. Such lack of blood supply causes heart attacks, strokes, high blood pressure, blindness, kidney failure, decreased walking capacity, and ulcers and gangrene of the feet and lower legs.

Life depends on an almost endless series of checks and balances of which the stickiness of our platelets is but one example. If our platelets couldn't stick together, we would *bleed to death.* But if they are too sticky, we would *clot to death.* What we want is the right balance.

Millions of people take an aspirin a day to reduce the stickiness of their platelets even though they don't know whether this is either necessary or effective for them. Studies at **The Hope Heart Institute** in Seattle, Washington, have shown that about 25% of people don't need aspirin because their platelets aren't sticky. The other 75% of people have sticky platelets. About 2/3 of these sticky platelet people have platelets that respond adequately to aspirin and 1/3 do not. The only way to find out who needs treatment to control excessive platelet aggregation and with what medication is to *do relevant tests.*

In addition to medications, the omega-3 fatty acids in fish and lignan-rich flaxseed oils (p. 282) reduce platelet stickiness.

3. Select a Good Doctor and Follow His or Her Advice

If your physician finds that you have a "genetic" cholesterol problem (such as a very high blood level of LDL with a family or personal history of coronary heart disease at age of 35 to 40 years), he or she may advise the Pritikin or the Ornish diet for you (p. 136). These diets limit calories from all types of fat to not over 10% of the total (*see* p. 141 for our preference).

If you retain fluid or have high blood pressure, your physician will request you to restrict salt. Of the salt you ingest, 90% is already in the packaged, canned, and fast foods you eat. Please read the labels and shop wisely.

Your physician may find that you need medications to decrease your blood pressure; lower your blood levels of LDL cholesterol, triglycerides, glucose, and homocysteine; and raise your blood levels of HDL cholesterol and omega-3 fatty acids. The highest sources of these essential fatty acids are lignan-rich flaxseed oil and fish oil (pp. 146, 282). Lignans (flaxseed fiber components) have antioxidant and anti-cancer properties.

You may need *magnesium* since most people are deficient in this essential mineral that steadies and strengthens the heart beat and decreases high blood pressure.

If you are a woman who has passed through menopause, your physician may advise you to take estrogens or other drugs to reduce your risk of developing osteoporosis (pp. 88, 287), possibly heart disease, and, perhaps, alzheimer's disease, too.

While medications are *not* substitutes for the five cardinal rules and the three additional strategies for heart-healthy (fit) living, they are very important additions when needed.

Section V:
Surgical Procedures

Surgical Procedures
for Arteries Irreversibly Damaged by
Atherosclerosis and its Complications

Two Types of Operations:
Vascular and Endovascular 202-211
Surgery to Increase the Blood Supply
   to the _Heart_ 212-227
   • Balloon Angioplasty for Single Coronary
      Obstruction 214
   • Balloon Angioplasty with
      Stent Placement 215
   • Single Coronary Bypass
      Using an Internal Mammary Artery 216
   • Balloon Angioplasty for
      Double Coronary Obstruction 217
   • Double Coronary Bypass
      Using Saphenous Vein Grafts 218
   • Double Coronary Bypass Using
      Internal Mammary Artery Grafts 219
   • Triple Coronary Bypass
      Using Saphenous Vein Grafts 220
   • Quadruple Coronary Bypass
      Using Saphenous Vein Grafts 221
   • Quadruple Coronary Bypass Using
      Three Saphenous Vein Grafts and One
      Internal Mammary Artery Graft 222
   • Quintuple Coronary Bypass Using
      Both Internal Mammary Arteries 223
   • Combined Coronary Bypass and
      Heart Valve Surgery 224-227

Surgery to Increase the Blood Supply to the _Brain_ and to Prevent Embolic Obstruction of Flow 228-229
- Carotid Endarterectomy 229

Surgery to Increase the Blood Supply to the _Kidneys_ 230-232
- Balloon Angioplasty and Stent Placement to Correct Narrowing of a Renal Artery 231
- Bypass Grafts to Renal Arteries 232

Surgery to Increase the Blood Flow to the _Legs_ 233-247
- Aortobifemoral Bypass 236
- Femorofemoral Bypass 237
- Axillofemoral Bypass 238
- Combined Axillofemoral and Femorofemoral Bypass 239
- Balloon Angioplasty of Left Common Iliac Artery 240
- Endarterectomy of the Arteries at the Groin 241
- Nature's "Operation" 242
- Balloon Angioplasty and Stent Placement of Distal Superficial Femoral Artery 243
- Above-Knee Femoropopliteal Bypass (Synthetic Graft) 244
- Below-Knee Femoropopliteal Bypass (Vein Graft) 245
- Femorotibial Bypass (Vein Graft) 246
- Femoropedal Bypass (Vein Graft) 247

Surgery for _Aortic Aneurysms_ 248-249
- Graft for Thoracic Aneurysm 248
- Graft for Abdominal Aneurysm 249

Two Types of Operations:
Vascular and Endovascular

The **need for surgery** to treat the complications of atherosclerosis **is an admission that prevention has failed** either because no program was followed, the program followed was inadequate, or the program was started too late. Whatever the reason, surgery is a vital backup for these patients. *But for optimal results, the best of surgical and medical care must be combined and continued for life.*

While surgery can literally accomplish wonders, we must not forget that all who are at risk to develop atherosclerosis and related clot formation need the preventive measures discussed in Sections III and IV. The "all who are at risk" includes nearly everyone in our affluent society. If the Five Cardinal Rules for heart-healthy (fit) living were followed, far fewer people would need operative help.

There are two very different types of operations that can be used to treat the abnormalities that occur in arteries as a result of atherosclerosis and clot formation. The first type is classified as **"open"** and the second as **"closed."**

The open type, called *vascular surgery*, exposes the arteries from the outside. This type of surgery uses endarterectomy procedures (Fig. 61, p. 204) and bypass grafts (Fig. 62, p. 204) for blockages, and inlay grafts (Fig. 63, p. 205) for aneurysms.

The closed type, called *endovascular surgery*, is done from inside the artery with devices brought to the diseased areas by long, slender, hollow tubes called catheters that are inserted through the skin into the arterial system with only a needle puncture (Fig. 64, p. 207). This new type of surgery is evolving rapidly (Fig. 65, p. 210; Fig. 66, p. 211).

Vascular Surgery
for
Obstructions and Aneuryms

Vascular surgery operations in general use today have been proven by time to be safe and reliable. Operations of this type are performed in well-lighted operating rooms by surgeons who make incisions through the skin and underlying tissues to expose the artery. The operations for obstructions usually involve opening the artery and removing the material that is blocking the lumen, a procedure called *endarterectomy* (Fig. 61, p. 204), or establishing a new pathway for blood to flow around the site of the blockage, a procedure called *bypass graft placement* (Fig. 62, p. 204). The operation for aneurysms involves replacing a weak tissue wall with a strong synthetic one, a procedure called *inlay graft replacement* (Fig. 63, p. 205).

Bypass Grafts for Obstructions

This procedure is accomplished by suturing one end of a graft to an opening made in the wall of the artery above the blockage and the other end to an opening made in the wall of the artery below the obstruction. The blood flows from the artery above the block through the graft into the artery below the obstruction.

Inlay Replacement Grafts for Aneurysms

The surgeon clamps the artery, usually the aorta in the abdomen, above and below the aneurysm, opens its front wall, removes the clot and debris (leaving the outer wall of the aneurysm intact), and then sutures a plastic graft to the inside of the aorta (artery) above and below the ballooned-out region to establish a secure inner channel with walls that won't rupture. The surgeon then trims the aneurysm sac and sutures its edges together, snugly encircling the graft with a layer of living tissue (p. 249).

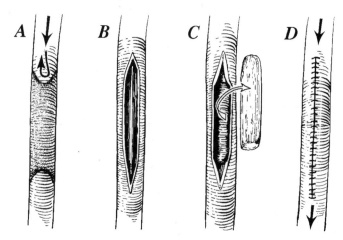

Figure 61 - Increasing the flow of red blood to the tissues by an endarterectomy procedure involves cutting into the artery, removing the material that is blocking the flow channel, and suturing the remaining wall back together.

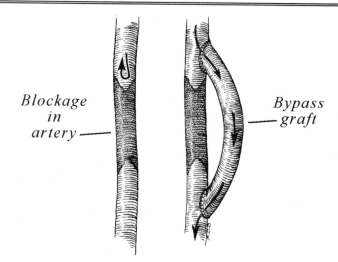

Figure 62 - Increasing the flow of red blood to the tissues by a bypass graft involves suturing one end of the graft to an opening made in the artery above the blockage and the other end to an opening made in the artery below the blockage.

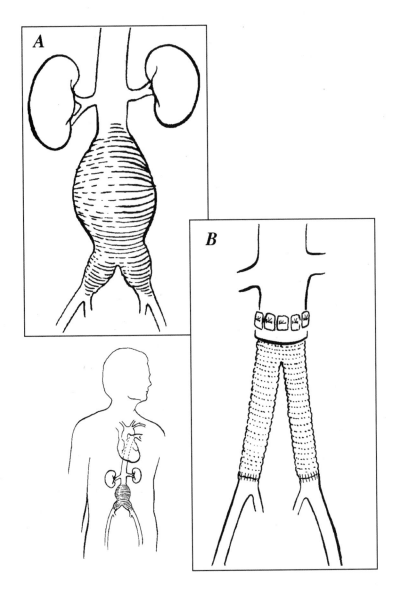

Figure 63 - Repair of an aneurysm of the abdominal aorta and common iliac arteries with a bifurcated Dacron graft to convey red blood to pelvis and legs. Wrapping of this inlay replacement graft with the outer layer of the aneurysm wall is not shown.

Endovascular Surgery
for
Obstructions

Endovascular surgical operations are procedures performed from within the blood channel with catheters inserted over guide wires introduced into the lumen of arteries, usually distant from the sites of blockage which require treatment. These catheters are advanced to the blocked areas under continuous x-ray visualization provided by monitor screens.

Catheters which have *inflatable balloons, cutting instruments,* or *grinding burrs* at their tips are used to remove obstructions. These operations are carried out in the semidarkness of space-age procedure rooms by cardiologists, radiologists, or vascular surgeons who precisely visualize what they're doing deep inside the body on monitor screens.

The operator begins these inside-the-artery operations by puncturing the skin, usually at the groin, with a needle that is advanced inward through the front wall of the underlying artery to enter the flow channel. The operator then passes a guide wire through the needle into the arterial channel and advances it upward or downward depending on the direction that the needle was inserted.

The operator then withdraws the needle, leaving the guide wire in place, and inserts a relatively large but short catheter, called a *sheath,* over the guide wire and advances it into the artery. The sheath has a *diaphragm* at its entrance through which guide wires and catheters can be introduced, withdrawn, and replaced without loss of blood. The sheath is like an on-off ramp to a superhighway (Fig. 64, p. 207).

When the operator has properly positioned the catheter,

Passage of Catheters into Arteries

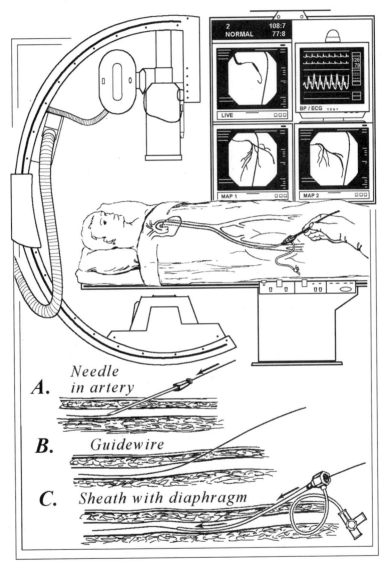

Figure 64 - Placement of a sheath into the big artery at the groin quickly establishes access into the arterial system and allows guide wires and catheters to be inserted, removed, and reinserted easily without loss of blood.

he/she withdraws the guide wire and advances the catheter to the desired location, such as into the coronary arteries. Next, the operator performs cineangiograms by injecting dye and taking films at a rapid rate to provide an x-ray movie of the flow of this fluid through the vessels.

In the case of a coronary artery, if an area of marked narrowing is discovered, the cardiologist passes a very thin, delicate guide wire with an exceedingly fine distal portion through the inserting catheter. The tip of this guide wire is so flexible that if it is pushed against the wall, the end will fold back on itself and produce no injury.

The cardiologist passes this fine guide wire through the site of narrowing and then advances a balloon-tipped catheter over it to center the deflated balloon across this site.

After checking to make sure that all is ready, the cardiologist inflates the balloon to high pressures that stretch and compress the wall and enlarge the lumen at the site of narrowing, a procedure called *Percutaneous Transluminal Coronary Angioplasty* (PTCA - Fig. 65, p. 210).

If the balloon result isn't good, the operator may repeat the procedure or advance a catheter with a burr or cutting device at its tip and grind or shave the obstruction away.

These balloon and other type procedures may tear the inner wall and partially detach a portion of it. If the fragment faces into the current, the flow force will drive it into the channel and block the blood path. To correct this problem, an ingenious, expandable, wire mesh device, called the *endovascular stent*, has been developed (Fig. 66, p. 211).

To deploy a stent, the operator passes a balloon-tipped

catheter that has a *contracted* stent positioned *over* the *deflated* balloon. The operator advances this catheter over the guide wire which had been had left in place after the initial dilation procedure.

In the case of a disrupted coronary artery, the cardiologist positions the balloon/stent across the site of blockage and *inflates* the balloon which *expands* the stent. The expanded stent *compresses* the separated layers of the coronary artery wall back together and *restores* an enlarged flow channel. The cardiologist then deflates the balloon and withdraws it, leaving the expanded stent in position which *maintains* the channel. The use of stents has extended the successful use of balloon angioplasty in the coronaries and elsewhere in the arterial system for the treatment of obstructions due to atherosclerosis and clot formation (p. 212).

Endovascular techniques have been developed for placing grafts inside **aneurysms** *to prevent these dilated areas from rupturing and causing fatal hemorrhage. Many aortic aneurysms in both the chest and abdomen can now be safely taken care of by these techniques. Further progress may be anticipated in this dynamic field which will expand the use of endovascular grafts for even more patients with aneurysms.*

Vascular and endovascular surgeons can now treat properly selected patients afflicted with diseased arteries caused by atherosclerosis and clots with relative safety and great benefit. Despite these remarkable advances, **our emphasis must remain on** *decreasing the need for operations of any type.* This can be accomplished by heart-healthy (fit) living begun in childhood and continued thereafter. Such a program would go a long way toward preventing atherosclerosis and its complications of blockage and aneurysm formation from developing as we age (p. 193).

Balloon Angioplasty

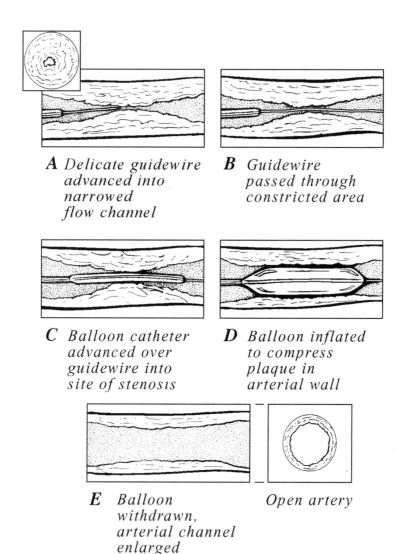

A *Delicate guidewire advanced into narrowed flow channel*

B *Guidewire passed through constricted area*

C *Balloon catheter advanced over guidewire into site of stenosis*

D *Balloon inflated to compress plaque in arterial wall*

E *Balloon withdrawn, arterial channel enlarged*

Open artery

Figure 65 - Balloon angioplasty is an endovascular operation that enlarges the narrowed flow channel of an atherosclerotic artery by inflating a balloon to dilate and enlarge the obstructed site.

Placement of Stent

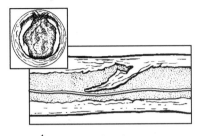

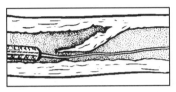

A *Detached portion
of arterial wall
blocks channel*

B *Deflated balloon
with contracted
stent advanced
over fine
guidewire*

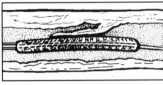

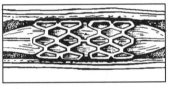

C *Balloon catheter
with stent moved
into place*

D *Balloon inflated,
stent expanded,
wall restored*

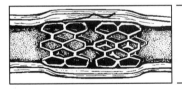

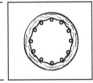

E *Deflated balloon
removed leaving
stent in place*

Open artery

*Figure 66 - Balloon angioplasty complicated by blockage of the
flow channel due to partial detachment of a portion of the wall.
This complication is corrected by expanding a contracted wire
mesh stent that compresses the separated layers back together,
holds them in position, and restores an enlarged flow channel.*

Surgery to Increase the
Blood Supply to the Heart Muscle

Last year about *900,000* operations (Figs. 67-78) were performed in the U.S. to increase the blood supply to the heart muscle at a cost of approximately $30 billion. About half of these operations were closed (endovascular) procedures performed by cardiologists using catheters with balloons or other devices, while the other half were performed by surgeons using open-heart techniques to place bypass grafts.

In general, *endovascular surgery* is best used for patients who have severe but localized obstructive disease of only one or two coronary vessels, while *vascular surgery* is best used to implant as many bypass grafts as needed for patients with severe obstructions of all their main coronary arteries.

The main advantages of the balloon (PTCA) procedures are that they require only a needle puncture, and the patients recover much faster than after open-heart operations. But there are two disadvantages, *acute closure* and *recurrent narrowing*.

Prior to the use of stents, (Fig. 66, p. 211) acute closure developed in 3 to 4% of patients. Now, with the use of stents, the frequency of this complication has been reduced to about 1%. But when it occurs, most of the patients must be rushed to the operating room for emergency placement of bypass grafts.

Prior to the use of stents, severe narrowing recurred after 3 to 6 months at the site of the balloon dilation in about 33% of the patients. With stents, this complication has been reduced to about 15%, and further improvements are expected. Most patients who develop severe recurrent narrowings will require additional procedures: some repeat balloon dilations, others dilations and more stents, and others bypass grafts.

Surgeons have most frequently used segments of the longest superficial vein in the leg to bypass blocked coronary arteries. About 50%, however, of these *greater saphenous grafts* develop severe atherosclerosis after 7 to 10 years and close off.

Fortunately, atherosclerosis rarely develops in the delicate *internal mammary arteries* that lie one on each side of the breastbone inside the front of the chest. These vessels have been superb when used as grafts to bypass blocked coronary arteries. At 10 years, 95% have been open with normal walls.

Because of these results, heart surgeons now use mammary grafts very frequently, including using them in "mini" operations to bypass blockages of the anterior descending branch of the left coronary artery. (Robotic surgery through keyhole openings is also in development.) Patients recover quicker from smaller operations done through short incisions without the use of the heart-lung machine.

The delicate gastroepiploic artery, which runs along the lower border of the stomach, also works very well as a graft to bypass obstructions of the coronary arteries.

The risk of mortality today for patients in good condition who must undergo either percutaneous transluminal coronary angioplasty (PTCA) or coronary artery bypass grafts (CABGs) for blockages of their coronary arteries should not exceed 1%.

The main drawback of standard coronary bypass graft surgery done with the heart-lung machine is that most patients need to convalesce for 6 to 8 weeks before they can return to full activity. But a strong recommendation for the bypass procedure is that even if the upper portions of all the main coronary vessels are severely blocked, excellent results maybe anticipated for many years in 90% of these patients.

Balloon Angioplasty for
Single Right Coronary Obstruction

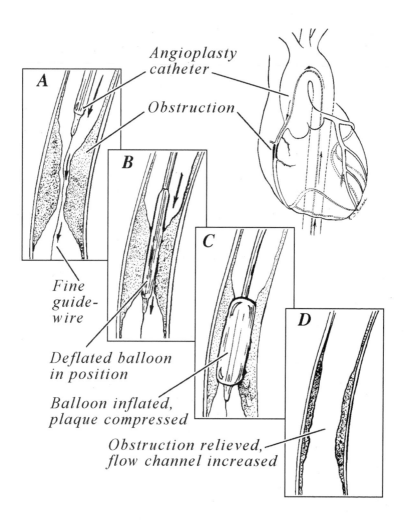

Angioplasty catheter

Obstruction

A

B

C

D

Fine guide-wire

Deflated balloon in position

Balloon inflated, plaque compressed

Obstruction relieved, flow channel increased

Figure 67 - Balloon angioplasty for severe stenosis (narrowing) of the upper mid-right coronary artery. This is the procedure of choice for most single and many double coronary artery blockages.

Balloon Angioplasty with Stent Placement

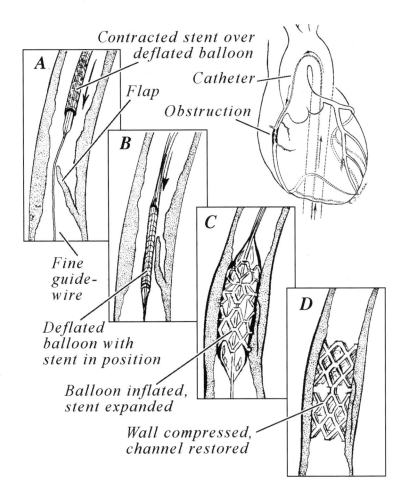

Contracted stent over deflated balloon

A

Flap

Catheter

Obstruction

B

Fine guide-wire

Deflated balloon with stent in position

C

D

Balloon inflated, stent expanded

Wall compressed, channel restored

Figure 68 - Use of wire mesh stent with balloon angioplasty for severe stenosis of the upper mid-right coronary artery. When balloon angioplasty partially detaches a segment of the wall, the dangling fragment will obstruct the flow channel if it faces into the current. Should this happen, use of a stent forces the layers of the wall back together, holds them in position, and restores an enlarged channel which converts a balloon failure into a success.

Single Coronary Bypass Using an
Internal Mammary Artery Graft
from Inside the Chest

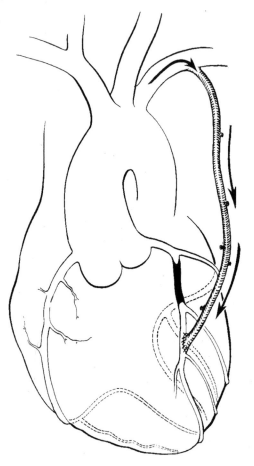

Figure 69 - Use of the left internal mammary artery to bring a new supply of red blood to the front of the heart when the upper anterior descending branch of the left coronary is completely blocked. This blockage is difficult to treat successfully by balloon angioplasty. In contrast, an internal mammary graft may be counted on to stay open indefinitely in this location under these conditions. Graft branches are closed by clips or bipolar cautery.

Balloon Angioplasty for Double Coronary Obstruction, One With and One Without a Stent

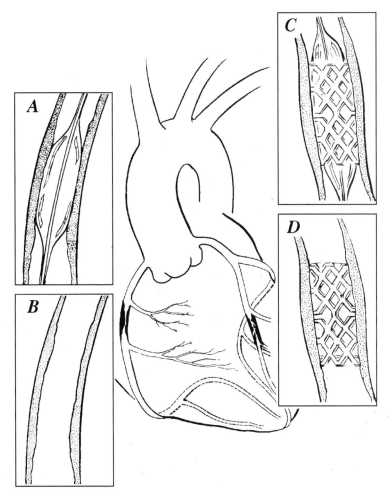

Figure 70 - Use of balloon angioplasty alone for an area of severe stenosis of the upper mid-right coronary artery, and use of balloon angioplasty with stent placement for severe stenosis of the upper midportion of the anterior descending branch of the left coronary artery. Stents are used in most PTCA procedures today.

Double Coronary Bypass Using Saphenous Vein Grafts from the Legs

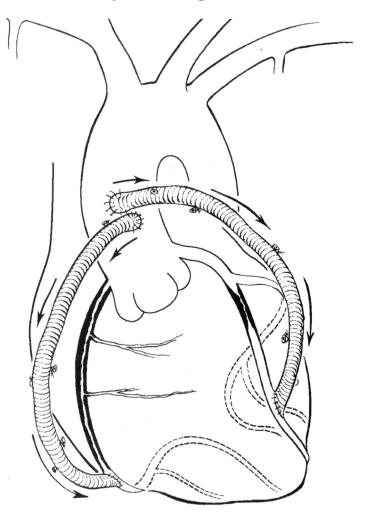

Figure 71 - Placement of two saphenous bypass grafts (superficial leg veins) from the aorta to the open coronary arteries beyond the severe obstructions brings new sources of red blood to supply the impoverished heart muscle. Branches of vein are tied off.

Double Coronary Bypass Using Both Internal Mammary Grafts

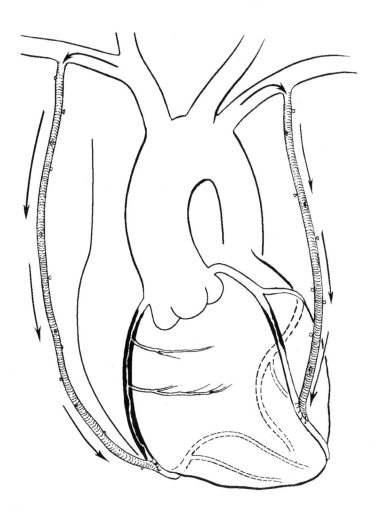

Figure 72 - Use of both internal mammary arteries to convey red blood to the same coronary sites shown in the previous figure, bypassing the areas of blockage. The advantage of using the internal mammaries is that they last longer than saphenous vein grafts; the disadvantage is that they are more difficult to use.

Triple Coronary Bypass Using Saphenous Grafts

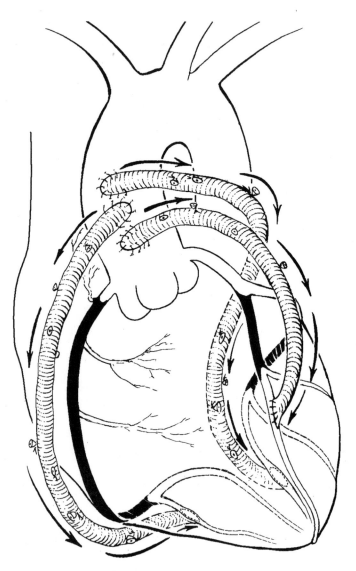

Figure 73 - Use of three saphenous vein grafts to convey red blood to three coronary sites, bypassing the areas of severe blockage.

Quadruple Coronary Bypass Using
Saphenous Grafts

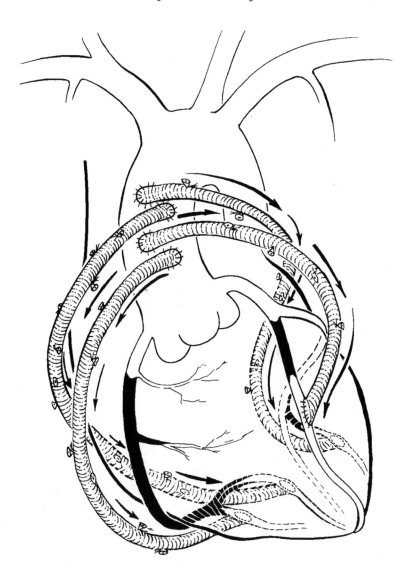

Figure 74 - Use of four saphenous vein grafts to convey red blood to four coronary sites, bypassing the areas of severe blockage.

Quadruple Coronary Bypass Using Three Saphenous Grafts and One Internal Mammary Artery Graft

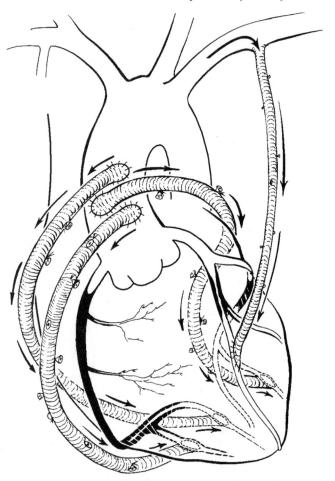

Figure 75 - Use of three greater saphenous vein grafts and the left internal mammary artery to convey red blood to four coronary sites, bypassing the areas of severe blockage. The left internal mammary is used for the most important vessel, the anterior descending branch of the left coronary. This bypass strategy is used frequently today.

Quintuple Coronary Bypass Using
Both Internal Mammary Arteries

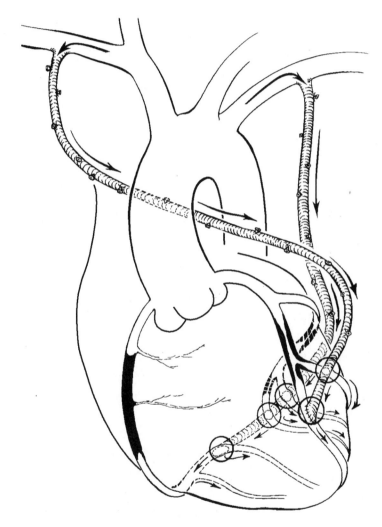

Figure 76 - Use of both internal mammary arteries to convey red blood to five coronary sites (circled), bypassing areas of severe blockage. This procedure is technically difficult, but it gives excellent long-term results.

Heart Valve Repair or Replacement in Conjunction With Surgery to Increase the Blood Supply to the Heart

Older patients who require surgery to increase the blood supply to their hearts may also need to have the function of their aortic and/or mitral valves improved (Figs. 77,78). If the openings of either of these valves are too small or leak (or both), the heart is in increased trouble. To pump the same volume of blood, the heart has to work harder when the valves don't work right. It's like a motor with gears grinding that is running out of gas. When both problems are fixed -- more fuel and well-functioning gears -- the motor hums. The heart is the same.

When our natural heart valves are functioning properly, they are a marvel of efficiency, moving swiftly in response to the pressure of the blood to open and close. Valves may become stiff and hard. When this happens, the diseased valve obstructs the flow of blood and forces the heart to do more pressure work. If valves leak, the heart has to do more volume work.

The most frequent mitral valve problem associated with decreased coronary blood supply to the heart is leakage. The decision to repair or replace the valve depends upon what the surgeon finds at the time of operation.

The most frequent aortic valve problem associated with decreased coronary blood supply is narrowing of the valve. The cusps of the aortic valve may become thick and stiff due to heavy scar tissue, and even rigid due to calcification. Such valves may also leak because their cusps can't close. In other patients, the problem may be purely leakage. When aortic valve surgery is required, the valve must nearly always be replaced because effective repair procedures are seldom possible.

There are several different types of valves that heart surgeons can use to replace their patients' diseased valves. Many are made of plastic and metal. Some are pig valves; others are human valves obtained from recently deceased accident victims.

Valves made from the tissue around the heart, the pericardium, of bovines also work well and are used frequently by heart surgeons.

In addition, in young patients the surgeon may replace the patient's diseased aortic valve with their own normal pulmonary valve and replace that valve with one removed from a recently deceased accident victim. This complex operation was developed by Dr. Donald Ross in England more than 30 years ago, and his first patient is still doing well.

Animal valves and valves made from other animal tissues are treated with chemicals to make them durable, flexible, and resistant to clot formation.

Because artificial (mechanical) valves are constructed of metal and plastic components, they tend to last longer than processed animal valves. But mechanical valves are more prone to have clots form on them than are tissue valves. Pieces of these clots may break off and be carried by the blood to the brain where they can produce a major stroke. Such free-floating fragments (emboli) block the blood flow when they plug an artery (p. 70; Fig. 33, p. 71; p. 280).

Clot formation can also impair the valve's function and necessitate emergency reoperation. Because of this, patients with mechanical valves are given drugs (usually Coumadin) to decrease the blood's ability to clot. This is seldom required for patients with tissue valves, especially those from humans.

Single Coronary Bypass and
Aortic Valve Replacement

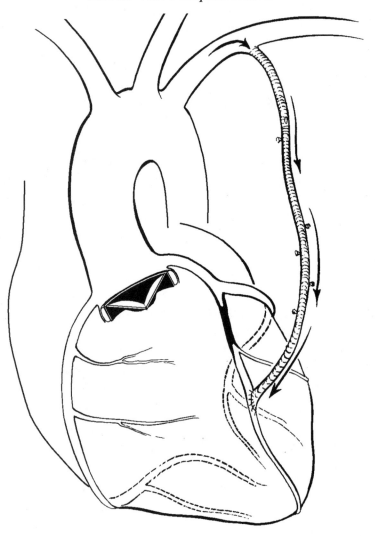

Figure 77 - Combined single coronary bypass using the left internal mammary artery to carry red blood to the anterior descending branch of the left coronary artery and aortic valve replacement with a St. Jude artificial heart valve (valve in closed position shown in cross section).

Double Coronary Bypass and Double Valve Replacement

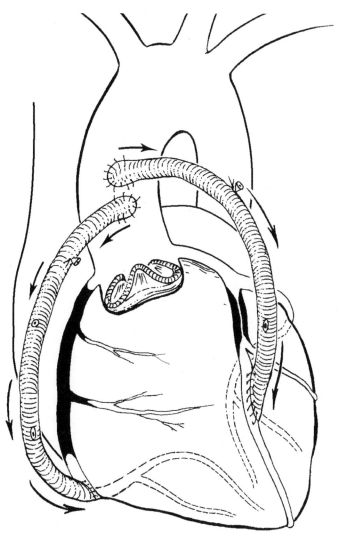

Figure 78 - Combined double coronary bypass (right and anterior descending branch of left) using two greater saphenous vein grafts and double valve replacement (aortic and mitral) with chemically processed pig valves.

Surgery to Increase
the Blood Supply to the Brain
and to Prevent
Embolic Obstruction of Flow

Carotid endarterectomy is the second most frequent arterial operation; the coronary bypass procedure is the most common.

Approximately 100,000 patients undergo carotid surgery each year in the United States for the purpose of preventing strokes. By far the most frequent operation performed for this purpose is carotid endarterectomy (Fig. 79), a procedure in which the surgeon removes the obstruction(s) and/or area(s) of ulceration that involve the division point (bifurcation) of the common carotid artery and the first portions (seldom over an inch) of the internal and external carotid arteries.

Platelet aggregates may form in the ulcerated areas (Figs. 33, 45; pp. 71,99). Fragments of these aggregates may break off and travel (embolize) into the vessels of the brain where they usually break up quickly and restore blood flow, producing only a *transient* ischemic attack (TIA -- Fig. 44, p. 98). Less often, hardening-of-the-artery debris may break away from the ulcerated area and go to the brain. These emboli tend to persist and cause permanent deficits.

Today, patients undergoing carotid endarterectomy are usually in the hospital for less than 24 hours, in contrast to several years ago when the average stay was 5 to 6 days. This shortened stay reduces the yearly health care costs for carotid surgery in the United States by about $300,000,000.

Carotid Endarterectomy

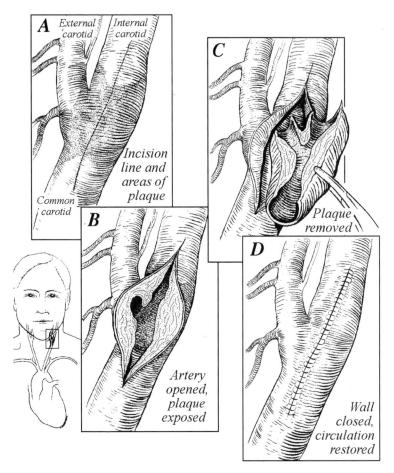

Figure 79 - The surgeon opens the obstructed division point of the common carotid artery, removes the diseased inner wall and any clot that is blocking the flow channel (the endarterectomy procedure), and sutures the outer wall back together to restore a full-caliber pathway with a smooth, glistening, clot resistant surface for the passage of red blood to the brain. This operation has been proven to be safe, effective, and long-lasting. Endovascular procedures have also been developed for this purpose, but cannot be recommended for general use at this time.

Surgery to Increase the Blood
Supply to the Kidneys

When the blood pressure is high because the blood supply to a kidney is low due a blocked renal artery, the vascular surgeon can restore a full supply of red blood to that kidney by either an endarterectomy or a bypass graft procedure.

Since the endovascular balloon-dilation surgery is also effective, this quicker, less invasive, closed technique has become "the operation" of choice for the initial treatment of renal artery blockages. Interventional radiologists perform most of these procedures.

The radiologist inserts the balloon catheter with a contracted stent from the groin, dilates the site of narrowing in the blocked renal artery, and leaves the expanded stent in position to maintain the enlarged flow channel (Fig. 64, p. 207; Fig. 80, p. 231). A few hours after the procedure is completed, the patient is discharged home and followed in the clinic.

Recurrent stenosis (narrowing) is the most common complication of the balloon dilation procedure. If stenosis recurs, it usually does so in the first 3 to 6 months, with about the same frequency as it does in the coronaries (15 to 20%, even with stents).

If severe blockage recurs with return of drug-resistant, high blood pressure, another endovascular procedure will usually be performed. Should the blockage recur again, placement of a bypass graft (or grafts) by a vascular surgeon may be necessary (Fig. 81, p. 232).

Balloon Angioplasty and Stent Placement to Correct Narrowing of a Renal Artery

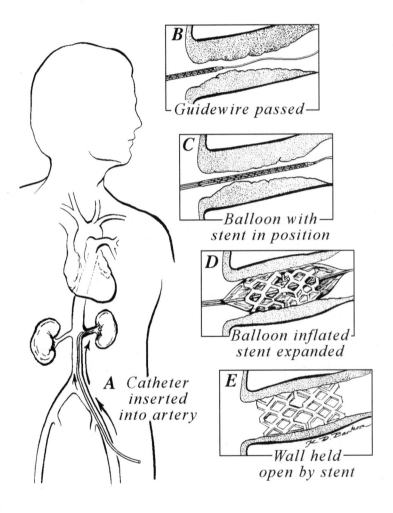

Figure 80 - This endovascular procedure is used for most cases of renal artery stenosis. The objectives of such surgery are to remove the obstruction, restore the blood flow to normal, decrease the elevated blood pressure, and preserve the function of the kidney.

Bypass Grafts to Renal Arteries

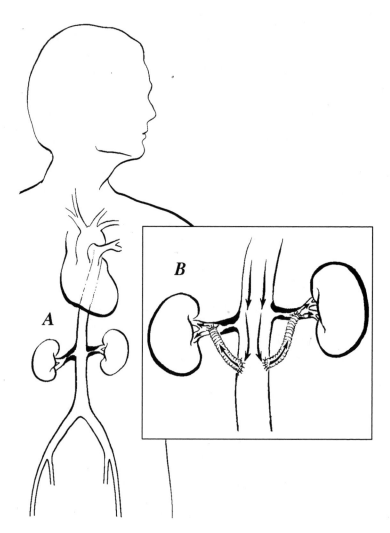

Figure 81 - (A) Bilateral stenosis of renal arteries. (B) Bypass grafts to renal arteries beyond the sites of obstruction carry red blood from the aorta to the kidneys, restoring flow, decreasing the elevated blood pressure, and preserving the function of the kidneys.

Surgery to Increase
the Blood Flow to the Legs

Obstruction of blood flow to the legs may occur from blockages of the arteries in the abdomen, at the groins, in the thighs, at the knees, and in the lower legs. These obstructions can occur at more than one site in the same patient and may be partial or complete. Both vascular and endovascular operations are important in their treatment (Figs. 82-93).

If surgery is to be done, the *patient's needs, general condition, and the extent of the blockages* determine which operation will be best for that patient. For obstructions of the abdominal aorta and/or the iliac arteries, vascular operations performed within the abdomen -- either to remove the thickened inner wall and clot or to implant synthetic grafts that bypass the blockages -- have proven to be reliable procedures to increase the blood supply to the legs.

When the iliac artery blood flow is good on one side and poor on the other, a synthetic graft can be placed to connect the leg arteries at the groin (common femorals), enabling the good side to supply red blood to the entire pelvis and both legs.

For high-risk patients whose iliac flow is low on both sides, a graft can be placed from the artery of an arm at the shoulder to the main artery of the leg at the groin on the same side and joined there to a graft which connects to the main artery in the other groin. This enables the main artery of one arm to supply red blood to the entire pelvis and both legs.

Today, many prefer the endovascular operations to reopen the blocked channels of the aorta and/or iliac arteries. This is accomplished by dilating narrowed sites with balloons, dissolving clots with drugs, and placing stents when needed.

If the thigh artery becomes blocked gradually as it runs from the groin to the knee, nature can usually build a satisfactory "bypass" of its own. Nature does this by developing collateral vessels between the profunda femoris and the popliteal arteries (Fig. 8, p. 21) which carry such a large amount of blood around the obstruction that the person can still lead a reasonably active life (Fig. 37, p. 81; Fig. 88, p. 242).

But there are some individuals whose collateral circulation isn't adequate and, if the blockage is over a few inches in length, placement of a bypass graft from the common femoral artery at the groin to the popliteal artery near the knee is the best way to restore circulation to the lower leg.

For shorter obstructions, endovascular operations employing balloons (often with stents) to open the arterial channel from the inside (Fig. 89, p. 243) have become accepted practice today even though the frequency of recurrent blockage is higher than that of bypass grafts made from the patient's veins.

If a surgeon implants an artificial graft to carry blood around an obstructed artery in the thigh of a patient who has sticky platelets that don't respond to aspirin or other medications, that graft will likely fill with clot after a few months and fail. For these patients, a vein taken from the patient's leg or arm should be used as the graft, because the blood flowing through it will not clot unless the flow becomes very slow.

But if an individual's platelets aren't sticky or can be made to become that way by medications (such as aspirin), that person's blood will likely be unable to clot off an artificial graft. In such patients, artificial grafts constructed of Dacron yarn or expanded Teflon can be used to bypass the occluded artery in the thigh with a high expectation of long-term success. The advantage of using artificial grafts under these circumstances is that the patient's greater saphenous and other veins can be saved to bypass obstructed arteries of the heart or lower legs, should this become necessary at a later time.

When the arteries below the knee are blocked in addition to those at the knee and in the thigh, the impairment of circulation to the foot is usually so marked that the patient is at high risk to lose the leg unless the circulation can be increased. In such circumstances, long-length grafts can often be placed from the big artery at the groin to a small artery near the ankle or even in the foot. **By far the best graft** for this demanding purpose is one of the patient's superficial veins, preferably the *greater saphenous* vein from a leg, or, as a second choice, an arm vein.

Endovascular operations are seldom applicable in the small vessels far below the knee, and, if attempted, are rarely successful. In fact, the closer to the foot a revascularization procedure has to be performed, the greater the necessity to use a healthy, living vein as the bypass graft. This is because the blood flowing through even the best of artificial grafts will clot long before it would in a natural vessel lined by healthy endothelial cells.

Sometimes procedures are required at two levels to adequately restore the blood flow to the lower extremities. Such combinations may involve two grafts -- for example, one graft placed from the big artery in the abdomen, the aorta, to the artery at the groin, the femoral, and another graft placed from there to the artery at the knee, the popliteal, bypassing obstructions in the abdomen and in the thigh. Endovascular and open vascular operations may also be combined -- for example, using a balloon angioplasty procedure to open a blocked common iliac artery in the abdomen and then using a graft from the common femoral artery at the groin to the popliteal artery at the knee to bypass the blocked thigh artery.

Aortobifemoral (Abdomen-to-Groin) Bypass

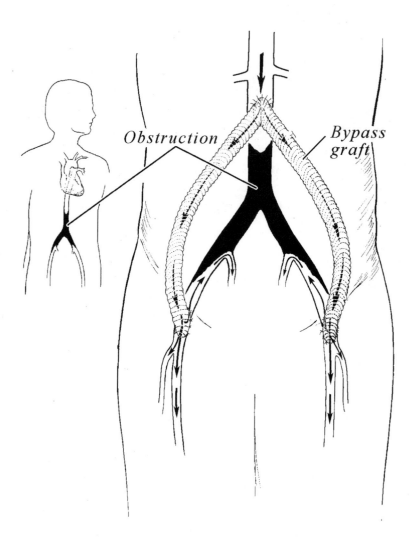

Figure 82 - Obstruction of the aorta and common iliac arteries blocks the flow of red blood to the pelvis and legs. A bypass graft from the aorta above the blockage to the femoral arteries below carries a new supply of red blood to the pelvis and the legs.

Crossover Femorofemoral (Leg-to-Leg) Bypass

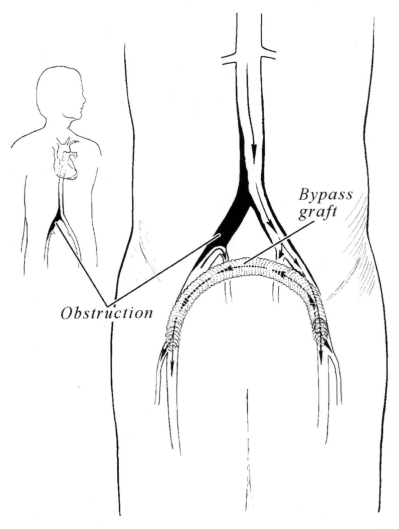

Figure 83 - In this instance, the right common iliac artery is closed, but the left is still adequately open to supply both sides. Placing a synthetic graft from the common femoral artery in the groin on the open side to the common femoral artery in the groin on the closed side enables the open side to supply red blood to the entire pelvis and both legs.

Axillofemoral (Arm-to-Leg) Bypass

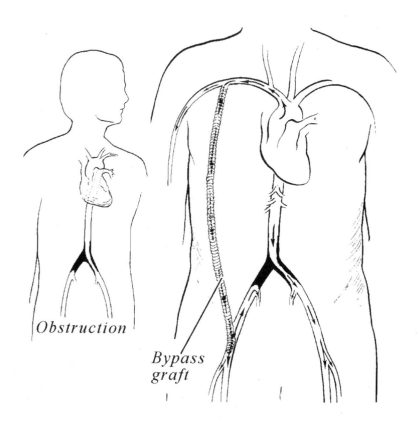

Obstruction

Bypass
graft

Figure 84 - Threatening decrease of the blood supply to the right leg due to complete occlusion of the right common iliac arteries in an elderly, fragile patient presents a problem when the blood supply to the left leg is too low to also supply the right leg through a leg-to-leg graft at the groin. Under these circumstances, diverting red blood to the common femoral artery in the right groin from the axillary artery going to the right arm through a graft called an "axillofemoral bypass" is an effective operation that the elderly patient can tolerate. The right leg gains much needed blood supply, and the supply of the right arm is not impaired.

Combined Axillofemoral (Arm-to-Leg) and Crossover Femorofemoral (Leg-to-Leg) Bypass

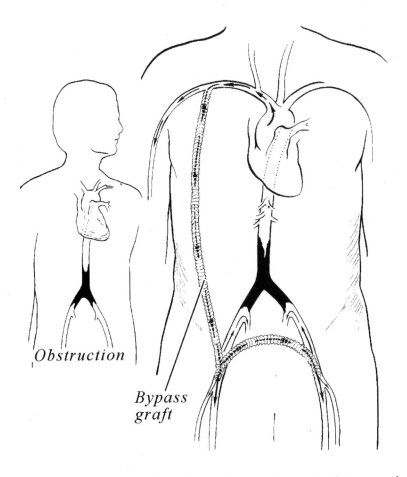

Figure 85 - For frail patients who are in need of increased circulation to the lower half of the body but can't tolerate a major vascular or endovascular operation within their abdomen, the combination of an arm-to-leg graft on one side with a leg-to-leg graft to the opposite side is an effective operation that relieves pain, avoids ulcers, heals small ones if present, and enables these fragile patients to walk within their limited general capacity. This procedure brings red blood to the entire pelvis and both legs.

Balloon Angioplasty with Primary Stent Placement for Narrowed Common Iliac Artery

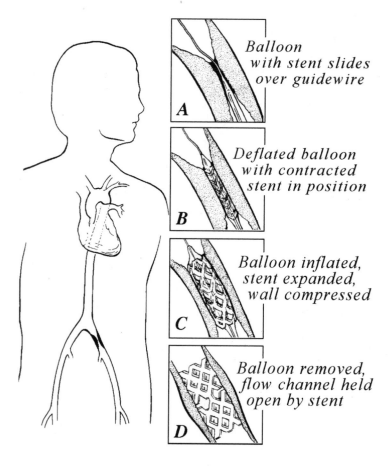

Balloon with stent slides over guidewire

A

Deflated balloon with contracted stent in position

B

Balloon inflated, stent expanded, wall compressed

C

Balloon removed, flow channel held open by stent

D

Figure 86 - Endovascular surgery using an inflatable, balloon-tipped catheter to dilate areas of narrowing in the common iliac arteries is now frequently followed by stent placement to compact the wall and expand the lumen. This procedure has largely replaced open vascular surgery (removal of the inner wall or placement of a bypass graft) for treatment of this lesion. Shown here is use of the balloon technique with primary stent placement to increase the flow of red blood to the pelvis and leg.

Endarterectomy of the Arteries at the Groin

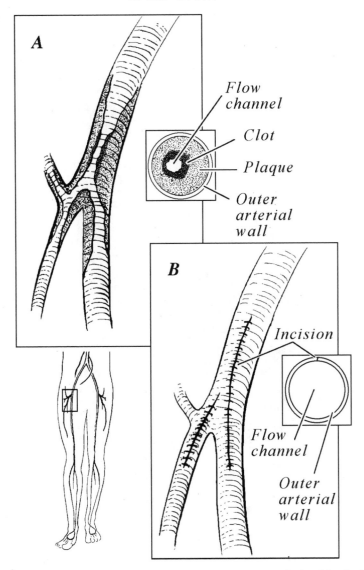

A

Flow
channel

Clot

Plaque

Outer
arterial
wall

B

Incision

Flow
channel

Outer
arterial
wall

Figure 87 - Endarterectomy (Fig. 61, p. 204) of the blocked arteries at the groin and upper thigh increases the flow of red blood to the thigh and lower leg.

Nature's "Operation" for Gradual Occlusion of the Thigh Artery

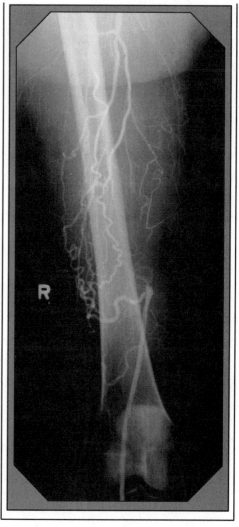

Figure 88 - As this patient's thigh artery became gradually blocked, such extensive collateral circulation developed between the profunda femoris and the popiteal arteries that it could supply enough red blood to the leg to support nearly full activity. Exciting new developments with gene therapy may enable nature to build bigger vessels faster, even in the heart.

Balloon Angioplasty with Primary Stent Placement for Narrowed Short Segment of the Lower Superficial Femoral (Thigh) Artery

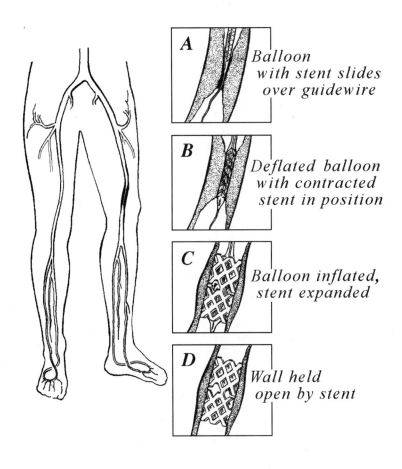

A Balloon with stent slides over guidewire

B Deflated balloon with contracted stent in position

C Balloon inflated, stent expanded

D Wall held open by stent

Figure 89 - Shown here is the use of the balloon technique with primary stent placement to open a short, narrowed segment of the main artery in the lower thigh.

*Groin-to-Above-Knee (Femoropopliteal) Bypass
Using a Synthetic Graft for
Long Segment Blockage of the
Superficial Femoral (Thigh) Artery*

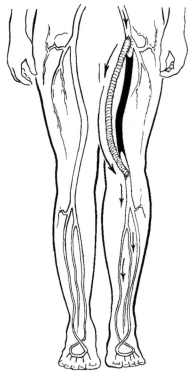

Figure 90 - Blockage of the superficial femoral artery in the thigh of a patient whose sticky platelets were made non-sticky by one regular aspirin a day. A bypass graft placed from the artery at the groin to the artery above the knee delivers needed red blood to the lower leg. A synthetic graft could be safely used in this patient because the patient's sticky platelets became much less sticky with aspirin. If the platelets hadn't changed, a vein graft would have been used instead. This patient will continue indefinitely to take one aspirin daily to keep his/her platelets from becoming sticky.

Groin-to-Below-Knee (Femoropopliteal) Bypass Using a Vein Graft for Long Segment Blockage of the Superficial Femoral (Thigh) and Upper Popliteal (Knee) Arteries

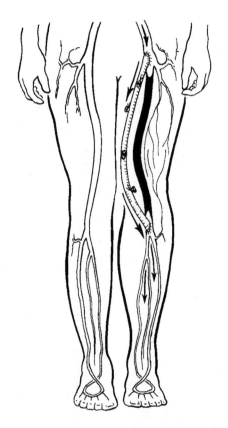

Figure 91 - Blockage of the superficial femoral and upper popliteal arteries severely impairs the supply of red blood to the lower leg. The greater saphenous vein (Fig. 29, p. 61) from this leg is placed as a graft from the artery at the groin to the artery below the knee. This graft conveys the needed red blood to the lower leg and is resistant to clot formation because of the healthy endothelial cells that cover its flow surface.

Groin-to-Lower-Leg (Femorotibial) Bypass Using a Long Vein Graft

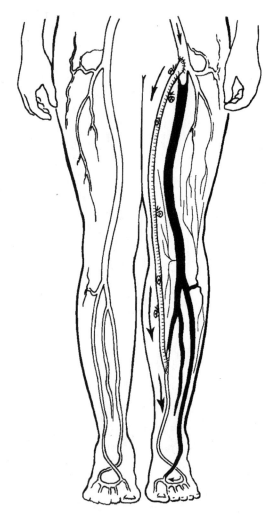

Figure 92 - Obstruction of the main leg arteries all the way to the foot except for one vessel in the lower leg. A long vein graft from the big artery in the groin to this open vessel provides an adequate supply of red blood to save the extremity and restore function.

Groin-to-Foot (Femoropedal) Bypass Using a Very Long Vein Graft

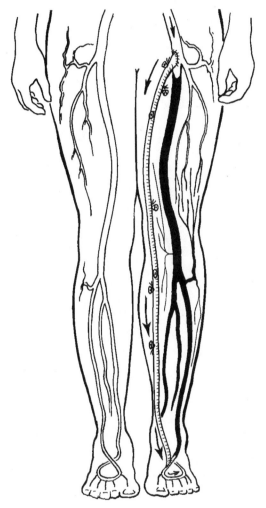

Figure 93 - Obstruction of the main arteries all the way to the foot critically impairs the blood supply to the lower leg and foot. Even so, in most cases, a very long vein graft from the big artery in the groin to a small artery in the foot provides an adequate supply of red blood to save the extremity and restore function.

Surgery for Aortic Aneurysms

The reason for removing an aortic aneurysm is to prevent fatal hemorrhage from rupture. In the most common technique, a synthetic graft is placed inside the outer wall of the aneurysm and sewn to the full thickness of the aortic wall above and below the ballooned-out segment. The remaining aneurysm wall is trimmed and then sutured to itself to form a tight tissue covering around the graft (Figs. 93, 94).

Inlay Replacement Graft for Thoracic Aneurysm

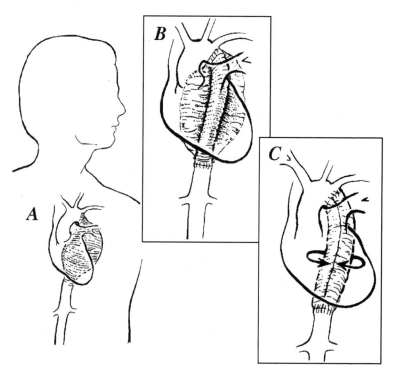

Figure 94 - (A) Life-threatening aneurysm of the aorta in the chest. (B) Aneurysm repaired by a Dacron graft placed inside the weakened and ballooned-out wall. (C) Outer wall of aneurysm sutured around graft. See page 209 for endovascular graft use.

Inlay Replacement Graft for Abdominal Aneurysm

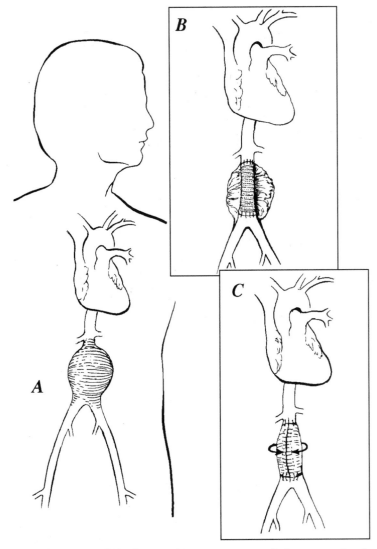

Figure 95 - (A) Life-threatening aneurysm of the aorta in the abdomen. (B) Aneurysm repaired by a Dacron graft placed inside the weakened and ballooned-out wall, preserving the aortic bifurcation. (C) Outer wall of aneurysm sutured around graft.

Section VI:

Related Heart Topics

- The Pacemaking and Conducting
  Systems of the Heart 251-253

- Artificial Pacemakers for the Heart 254-257

- Cardiopulmonary Resuscitation (CPR) 258-260

- The Automatic Internal Cardiac Defibrillator 261-263

- Heart Transplantation 264-266

The Pacemaking and Conducting Systems of the Heart

The pacing system of the heart is made up of special cells that build up an electric charge -- discharge it over the conducting system -- build up another charge -- discharge it -- and continue to do this indefinitely. The cells that fire fastest set the rate of the heartbeat (Fig. 96, p. 252).

The electrical impulses that originate from the pacemaking cells spread over the special pathways of the conducting system to reach the muscle cells of the heart and cause them to contract in a coordinated manner that enables the right ventricle to pump the blue blood to the lungs and, at the same time, the left ventricle to pump the red blood to the rest of the body.

The pacing cells that fire fastest are in a structure called the *sinus node*, which is located in the top portion of the front wall of the right atrium where the superior vena cava enters to return the blue blood from the upper part of the body. With sedentary activity these cells build up and discharge an electrical impulse about 80 times a minute to drive the heart. During exercise these cells discharge at a faster rate; during sleep they discharge at a somewhat slower rate.

If the sinus node cells lose their pacing ability, the next cells further along in the pacing system take over at their slower rate. Then, if these cells lose their pacing ability, the next cells down the line take over, etc., the pulse rate becoming progressively slower as this happens.

The Pacemaking and
Conducting Systems of the Heart

Sinus node

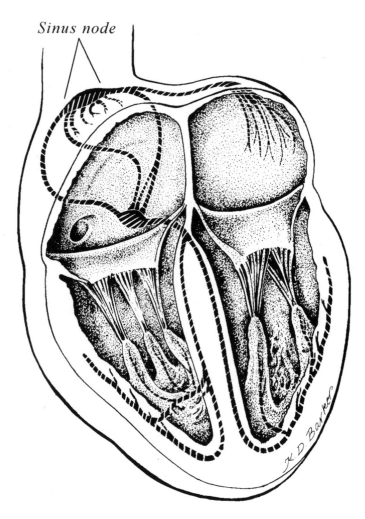

Figure 96 - Normally, the electrical impulses that cause the heart to contract arise in the sinus node and spread from there in an orderly sequence to cause the atria to beat first and then the ventricles.

Sometimes when the sinus node cells lose their ability to pace the heart, the beat becomes so slow that the decreased circulation causes the patient to become weak and dizzy. The heart may even stop. If it stops for more than 10 seconds, the patient loses consciousness because the brain's tiny oxygen reserve is used up so fast.

Fortunately, when this happens, the cells of the sinus node or of some other site further down the pacing system will generally start firing within 15 to 20 seconds, restoring the heart beat and the circulation. With the return of circulation, the brain receives oxygen and glucose and quickly regains its function. Within seconds the patient awakens with no recollection of having been unconscious.

When the heart stops, there is always danger it may not start again or that it may start too late. If the heart stops for four or more minutes, the lack of oxygen during the arrest period irreparably damages the brain cells.

Malfunction of the pacing and conduction system of the heart affects millions of people worldwide. Prior to the development of the early pacemakers in the 1950s, these difficult and often deadly problems could only be treated by medicines that were usually ineffective.

The conductive system of the heart is indeed a marvel of design and function. The sinus node sets the pace of the heart like the conductor of a symphony sets the tempo of the orchestra. The beat of the heart is the *music of life*.

Artificial Pacemakers
for the Heart

Artificial pacemakers have been developed to treat patients who can't function normally because their heart rates are too slow or who are in danger of death from their hearts stopping. Pacemakers consist of two main components: a miniaturized battery (pulse generator) with electronic sensing and firing mechanisms packaged in a metal container and one or two electrodes with long leads. Each electrode with its attached lead is inserted into a vein and advanced into the right side of the heart where it attaches to the inner wall. The other end of the lead is inserted into the connecting port of the pulse generator (Fig. 97, p. 255; Fig. 98, p. 257).

After these connections are completed, the pulse generator is placed beneath the fatty layer of the anterior chest wall a short way below the collarbone. The attachment of the lead or leads to the heart on one end and to the pulse generator on the other end enables this unit to monitor the electrical activity of the heart and, when necessary, to serve as its pacemaker. This function is painless to the patient who is unaware when the artificial pacemaker is firing.

When the pacemaking cells discharge an impulse and cause the muscle cells to contract, electric currents are generated. The electrocardiogram (ECG) is a record of these electrical events. The electrode(s) attached to the inner surface of the heart transmits a continuous ECG back over the lead(s) to the sensing mechanism in the pulse generator. This mechanism monitors the heart's action, and if the beat slows to the preset level for firing, the generator discharges electric impulses that travel rapidly over the lead(s) to the electrode(s) from whence these impulses spread to the muscle cells throughout the heart and stimulate them to contract.

Artificial Ventricular Pacemaker for the Heart

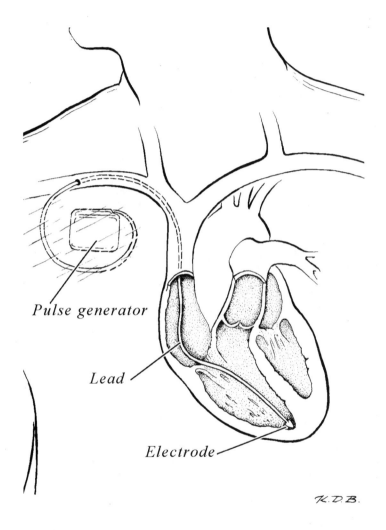

Pulse generator

Lead

Electrode

K.D.B.

Figure 97 - A single electrode is positioned in the right ventricle where it monitors the electrical activity of the heart, and if the heart rate falls below the pacemaker's setting, the pulse generator fires at its preset rate and stimulates the ventricles to contract.

These electronic units can be programmed to keep the heartbeat from dropping below any rate that is selected. For example, if the activation rate of the pacer is set at 50, and the patient's heart rate drops below 50, the pacer senses this immediately and begins firing at its preset rate of 50 times a minute. Each time the pacer fires, the heart contracts in response to the electrical impulse and pumps blood to the lungs and body. The pacer is now the heart's pacemaker. When the patient's natural heart rate again becomes faster than that of the pacer, the pacer returns to its "sensing" only mode and waits -- ever ready to be called into action.

Today, there are many sophisticated pacemakers that function so superbly that they are able to effectively treat nearly all of the pacing problems that patients experience. Many modern pacemakers have two leads, one that is positioned in the right atrium and one in the right ventricle. With these leads, the pacer is able to monitor the electrical activity of both the atria and the ventricles and pace them to function in a normal, integrated manner when called on to do so.

Some pacemakers are activity-responsive and fire faster when the patient exercises and slower when the patient rests.

Implanting a pacemaker is usually an easy procedure done under local anesthesia. These amazing devices have now been implanted in millions of patients worldwide. Last year approximately 120,000 pacemakers were implanted in the United States alone. Most of these units are warranted by the manufacturers for five years, but today many are expected to last 10 or more years before the pulse generator will need to be changed. Changing the generator is a simple operation done with local anesthesia in outpatient surgery.

Artificial Combined Atrial and Ventricular Pacemakers for the Heart

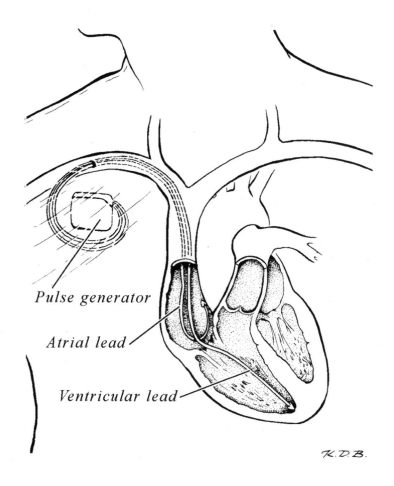

Pulse generator

Atrial lead

Ventricular lead

K. D. B.

Figure 98 - This pacemaker with two electrodes, one positioned in the right atrium and the other in the right ventricle, stimulates the atria to contract first and then the ventricles in a normal time sequence. The output of the heart with this type of pacemaker is significantly higher than with pacemakers that pace only the ventricles.

Cardiopulmonary Resuscitation (CPR)

When the heart stops, cardiopulmonary resuscitation (CPR) is the emergency procedure employed to get the circulation going again before the most sensitive organ, the brain, is damaged by lack of oxygen. Circulatory stoppage for as short a time as four minutes will cause severe brain damage. For people whose hearts stop, their survival depends largely on how quickly they are found and what the first person who finds them does (Fig. 99).

The heart may stop in one of two ways. It may suddenly cease beating and lie still, showing no motion. This type of stoppage is called *cardiac arrest*. More commonly, when the heart stops beating, it develops a wiggling type of uncoordinated motion that is unable to pump blood. This type of stoppage is called *ventricular fibrillation*.

To be successful, CPR must get oxygen into and carbon dioxide out of the blood and then pump this life-giving fluid to the tissues where it sustains them until the heart regains its beat and the patient is breathing again in an adequate manner. In the usual case of heart stoppage that occurs outside the hospital, the person performing CPR alternately ventilates the lungs by mouth-to-mouth respiration and then pumps this refreshed blood (replenished with oxygen and depleted of carbon dioxide) to the tissues by pushing the lower portion of the breastbone (sternum) inward to compress the heart.

If one day you should hear a thud in the adjacent room, and on investigation find that someone, perhaps your husband or wife, has collapsed, is unconscious, isn't breathing, and has no pulse, quickly pick up the phone and dial 911. Tell the attendant what's wrong and ask the medics to come

Cardiopulmonary Resuscitation (CPR)
Single Rescuer

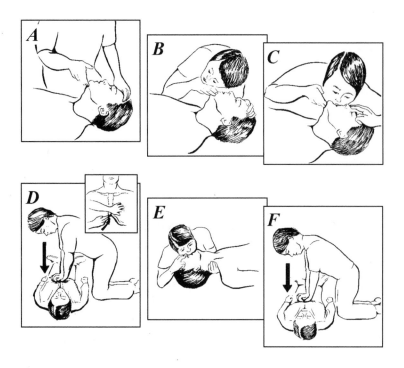

Figure 99 - (A) After giving a strong thump to the chest over the heart, tilt the patient's chin up and rotate the head back to hold the airway open. (B & C) If the patient still isn't breathing and has no pulse, pinch the nose shut and give two deep mouth-to-mouth breaths (1 to 2 seconds per breath) while holding the airway open. (D) Then compress the lower sternum sharply inward 15 times at a rate of about one compression every 2/3 of a second (Sternal compression also provides some pulmonary ventilation.). (E & F) Continue this "breathe and compress" sequence until the heart is beating and the patient is breathing or until help arrives to relieve you. CPR can be continued for an hour or even more with complete recovery in favorable circumstances.

immediately to your address. *It's valuable to **practice** this **call**, because in an emergency any of us can mentally block and forget 911, our phone number, and even our address. Try it now! When it's for real, **seconds count.***

Then quickly turn the patient on his/her back, and lift the chin up with one hand while rotating the forehead back with your other hand to extend the neck. This moves the lower jaw forward and lifts the tongue and epiglottis away from the back of the throat to open the airway. Now follow the "breathe and compress" sequence given in Fig. 99, p. 259.

If two people are available to resuscitate the patient, one tends to the lungs and the other to the heart. In this situation, the person tending to the breathing gives one big breath over about two seconds and then waits while the person tending to the heart gives five sternal compressions at a rate of about one every 2/3 second. The two-person team continues this 5:1 cycle until professional help arrives or the patient's heartbeat and breathing have returned.

The arrested heart will often begin to beat after starting CPR, but this doesn't happen with heart stoppage due to ventricular fibrillation. The fibrillation must be stopped first, and this must await the arrival of the emergency medical technician team in response to your 911 call. Generally, the team arrives within minutes to take over CPR. If the heart is fibrillating, the medics will get the heart in the best possible condition before shocking it with an electric current from a *defibrillator* to stop the fibrillation. CPR is continued, awaiting for the heart to begin beating.

After the heart is beating again, the patient is taken to an appropriate hospital for intensive care and later investigation to determine what caused the heart to stop and what can be done to prevent it from stopping again.

The Automatic Internal Cardiac Defibrillator (AICD)

An automatic internal cardiac defibrillator (AICD) is like a pacemaker, only its battery is bigger and more powerful, and its electronic sensing and firing mechanisms are programmed to detect and treat ventricular fibrillation rather than a slow heart rate (Fig. 100, p. 262).

Several years ago, two electrodes and leads were required to defibrillate the heart, and they were so big that the chest had to be opened to place them on the outside of the heart. Today, only one lead is needed, and its electrode has been made sufficiently small that it can be inserted into a vein -- like the lead of a pacemaker -- and advanced into the right side of the heart where it attaches to the inner wall of the right ventricle. The other end of this special lead is inserted into the connecting port of the pulse generator. This unit is then placed beneath the fatty layer of the anterior chest wall a short distance below the collarbone in a similar position to that employed for the smaller pulse generator of a pacemaker.

Automatic internal cardiac defibrillators have now been implanted in hundreds of thousands of patients around the world who are at high risk of sudden death from their hearts developing ventricular fibrillation. Because the ventricles are the main pumping chambers of the heart, when they arrest or fibrillate, the circulation stops.

Typically, a patient with an implanted defibrillator whose heart arrests or fibrillates begins to feel faint within a few seconds of the stoppage and would soon fall to the floor unconscious if it were not for activation of the defibrillator electrode attached to the heart. The sensing mechanism of the unit diagnoses what is wrong and quickly treats it.

The Automatic Internal Cardiac Defibrillator (AICD)

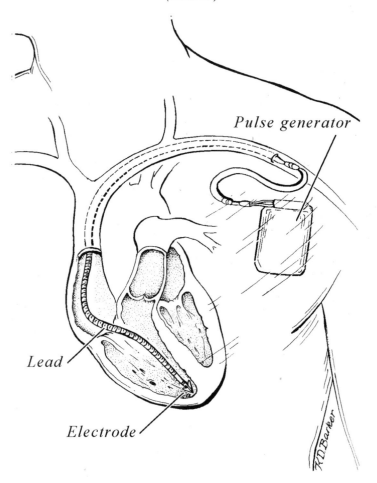

Figure 100 - The automatic internal cardiac defibrillator (AICD) monitors the electrical activity of the heart, and if ventricular fibrillation occurs, the generator discharges a strong electrical impulse that shocks the heart and stops the fibrillation. Usually the heart quickly regains its beat, but if it does not, the generator paces the ventricles like a pacemaker.

If the heart has arrested, the pulse generator of the AICD unit discharges an appropriate impulse that paces the heart like a conventional pacemaker. If the sensing mechanism detects that the ventricles are fibrillating, the pulse generator discharges a stronger impulse that stops the fibrillation.

After a few seconds, the still heart usually starts to beat. But if it does not, the sensing mechanism recognizes this and activates the pacing cycle.

With the return of the heart beat, the circulation begins to deliver oxygen and glucose to the brain. As this happens,the patient's sense of faintness disappears. When the heart is beating on its own at an adequate rate, the AICD unit returns to its "sensing only" mode.

There is no question that further major technologic advances may be expected in this dynamic field. Recent developments include pacemaker-AICD combinations and implantable defibrillators for atrial fibrillation which affects millions of people. Atrial fibrillation is a condition in which the atrial contractions are ineffective, discoordinated, irregular, and usually very fast. The ventricles beat in an irregular manner, too fast in some patients and too slow in others. Even so, most patients do reasonably well even though the output of their hearts is reduced 10 to 20%. The greatest danger of atrial fibrillation is clot formation in the left atrium with embolization of a clot fragment to the brain, causing a stroke. Anticoagluant drugs, most often Coumadin, are used to prevent this from occurring.

Heart Transplantation

Heart transplantation has become an excellent treatment for patients whose hearts are worn out and can't be repaired. But the main factor limiting greater use of this operation is the small number of donor hearts that are available. In the United States there are **only** about **2,500 donor hearts** that are suitable for transplantation which become available **each year**. The demand is much greater. Tens of thousands die for lack of a donor heart. A permanent artificial heart is needed.

The best donor hearts come from young accident victims with healthy hearts whose brain function has been destroyed by massive head injuries. If the family consents to their loved one's organs being used for the benefit of others, the donor's body is kept alive on a respirator for a few days while tissue matches are established with potential heart, lung, liver, kidney, pancreas, and small intestine transplant recipients who are usually within 500 miles of the donor's location.

We shall now comment specifically about transplantation of the human heart.

When all the arrangements for the heart transplant have been made, the procurement team from the recipient's center flies to the donor's city and removes the brain-dead donor's beating heart. The heart is rinsed free of blood, cooled to 4°C, and kept at that temperature while the team flies back to deliver the cold, pale, limp heart to the implant team in the operating room where the recipient is ready to be placed on bypass using the heart-lung machine.

It's now **"Go!"** The surgical team moves rapidly. Bypass is begun. The patient's old, sick heart is removed and the donor's new, healthy one is sutured in its place (Fig. 101).

Heart Transplantation

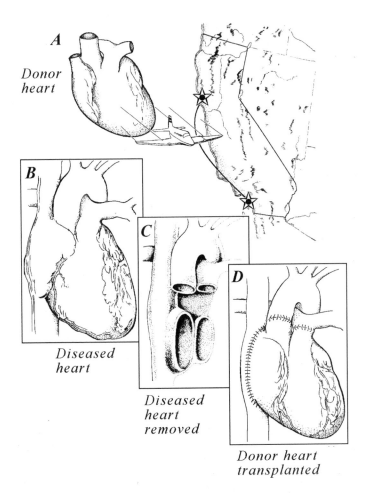

Figure 101 - In this case, the procurement team from Los Angeles flies to San Francisco and removes the heart from a brain-dead donor. This team flies back to Los Angeles and delivers the heart to the implant team waiting in the operating room. The surgical team then proceeds rapidly to place the patient on heart-lung bypass, remove the recipient's worn-out heart, and implant the donor's healthy heart in its place.

With the new heart sutured in position, the decisive moment has now arrived -- the clamp is removed from the patient's aorta. The unspoken question, "Will the heart beat?" is foremost in everyone's mind as the warm, red blood flows into the coronary arteries and begins to return color, warmth, and function to the transplanted heart.

As the blood surges through the coronaries, the heart becomes pink and often without an electric shock suddenly starts to beat and restores the *pulse of life*.

As this happens, all in the operating room breathe a sign of relief and thank God for answering their silent prayers.

As the heart gains strength, the surgeon directs the perfusionist running the heart-lung machine to progressively transfer the pumping of blood to the new heart. When the heart is doing all the work, the patient, now completely dependent on the transplant, begins a new life with the donor's gift at the center of his or her physical being.

After the wound bleeding has been stopped, the surgical team closes the chest. Then, when the anesthesiologist is satisfied with the patient's condition, the patient is taken to the cardiac intensive care unit. Within a short time, the patient awakens and the *miracle of life continues*.

Today, about 80% of the patients who received a heart transplant five years ago are doing well. Fifteen years ago, such results were but a dream. The research of yesterday made this advance possible by discovering safer and more effective drugs to prevent the patient's immune system from rejecting the donor's heart. Research yet to be done will make tomorrow's results even better.

Section VII:

Spiritual Reflections

It is fitting to conclude this book about the physical structure and function of our intricate human bodies by pausing to reflect on the spiritual aspects of our eternal lives. We are more than mere matter; we are body and soul, created by God for all eternity. It is appropriate, therefore, that we each seek inspiration for maintaining the health of our mortal bodies by also considering the vitality of our immortal souls.

We suggest that as strength and vigor are hallmarks of robust physical health, peace and joy are indications of **vibrant spiritual well-being**. There is now no doubt that such a spiritual state **has a positive influence on our physical condition**. God gives this joyful state to us when we serve those who need us out of our open hearts in a spirit of love.

Although most of us feel quite comfortable talking and thinking about the importance of taking good care of our physical bodies, it is rare that we stop to assess our spiritual status. As a result of failing to do this, we tend to merely exist rather than truly live. Though there is real mental work in pausing to face this vital issue, the reward is worth the effort. The appreciation of our life's purpose, value, and spiritual destiny is at stake. And further, our happiness,

"... that priceless peace of mind, serenity of soul, and exhilaration of spirit ... ,"

depends on what we do in response to this appreciation.

A powerful attraction of all the great religions is the simplicity of the means they advocate for obtaining happiness -- loving one's neighbor as oneself. Love in this context may, perhaps, best be defined as the freely giving of self for the benefit of another.

Christ set the example of love for humankind by becoming one of us in a stable at Bethlehem and in dying for us on a cross atop Calvary. He gave us clear direction when He said, "Whatsoever you do unto the least of these, you do unto Me." The world's other great religions -- including Judaism, Hinduism, Buddhism, and Islam -- all convey similar messages. They teach in different yet similar ways that a life barren of love is devoid of real meaning and true happiness.

In this context, we should see ourselves broadly as members of one worldwide human family, even though we may profess different religions and live distant from one another. Each of us in our own unique way can become an increasingly effective instrument of God's ministry to all people by serving those in need out of love.

The call to serve God by serving each other out of love is ever before us. We will all find purpose, worth, and happiness in our lives if we answer this call. And if we don't, we shall perish. There are no other options. It seems an easy choice.

The holy scriptures of all the major religions come together in their teaching that each of us is unique in our own way, and that **there is a divine purpose for every human life**. And that divine purpose is to love and serve God by serving each other out of love. God waits within our soul for us to find and follow Him on this path of human service. When we do, God rewards us with that pristine state of consciousness in which we experience peace, joy, and happiness.

Through the perspective of medicine, as in no other field of human endeavor, our lives are clearly seen to be time limited. We are awed by the realization that there must be **something greater than ourselves** which is responsible for our human existence and everything around us.

In preparing this book, we have felt the wonders of the physical marvel and spiritual essence that comprise us all. In reading this book, we hope you have felt this, too.

Our progress through life and the degree of happiness we derive from this journey to eternity and what we'll find when we get there will be largely determined by the road we travel in this life. Will it be the way of hatred, envy, greed, and anger or the less traveled route of love, joy, peace, and compassion? The choice is ours.

To obtain the priceless treasures of spiritual peace and joy, we must first see God in the soul of every human being, including ourselves. Gandhi said, *"If you don't see God in the next person you meet, it's a waste of your time to look further."* Only when this has become reality to us will we be able to follow the requests of the Holy Spirit to **"Tend My flock and feed my sheep"** *by helping those in need out of love.* By serving God through serving humanity, we will be fulfilling our destiny and achieving our full spiritual potential.

Mother Teresa said, "It's not how much we do that matters, but how much love we put in what we do that counts with God." To do this is the ultimate challenge and true adventure of our lives. By her life, Mother Teresa invites us to live our lives by traveling the road of service for those who need us. In this exciting journey, our days will overflow with happiness. **We cannot ask for more.**

To conclude this section, let us take the immortal words of St. Francis of Assisi into our hearts as we continue our earthly journeys to eternity:

Prayer of St. Francis

Lord, make me an instrument
of your peace.

Where there is hatred,
let me sow love;
Where there is injury, pardon;
Where there is doubt, faith;
Where there is despair, hope;
Where there is darkness, light;
And where there is sadness, joy.

O Divine Master, grant that I may not
so much seek to be consoled as to console;
to be understood as to understand;
to be loved as to love.

For it is in giving that we receive,
it is in pardoning that we are pardoned,
and it is in dying
that we are born to eternal life.

Section VIII:

Glossary

Aneurysm - An arterial segment that has ballooned (bulged) out because its wall has become weak due to disease or injury. The bulging occurs because the pressure of the blood within the flow channel stretches the weakened wall. Aneurysms are most common in the big artery in the abdomen, the aorta. The wall of an aortic aneurysm will usually continue to stretch until the pressure of the blood within it eventually ruptures the wall and causes massive hemorrhage, necessitating high-risk emergency surgery.

Angina Pectoris - Pain felt in the left anterior chest wall due to an insufficient supply of oxygenated (red) blood to the heart muscle.

Anticoagulants - Drugs which delay clotting of the blood (coagulation). When given in cases where a blood vessel is plugged up by a clot, anticoagulants act to prevent new clots from forming and existing clots from enlarging, but they don't dissolve clots. Coumadin and heparin are anticoagulants.

Antioxidants - Chemicals that neutralize atoms (mainly oxygen atoms) that have lost electrons from their outer orbits. Such atoms are referred to as "oxidized" or "oxygen free radicals." These radicals injure neighboring tissues by robbing them of electrons. New evidence suggests that the oxidized form of LDL cholesterol is the chemical that damages the arterial wall.

Aorta - The biggest artery in the body. It arises from the outlet of the left side of the heart and arches up above it like the handle of a cane that is directed to the back and left side of the chest near the midline. The aorta then passes downward through the back of the chest and abdomen, coming to lie in front of the spine in the lower portion. The aorta gives off many branches which carry blood to all parts of the body. At the level of the umbilicus, the aorta divides into the right and left common iliac arteries which descend to supply their side of the pelvis and the leg below.

Aortogram - An x-ray examination of the aorta made after injecting dye into the blood that shows the flow channel of this large vessel and its branches.

Arrhythmia - Variation from the normal rhythm of the heartbeat.

Arteries - The vessels that carry blood away from the heart. The pulmonary arteries convey the deoxygenated (blue) blood pumped out by the right ventricle to the lungs where it takes up oxygen, gives off carbon dioxide, and becomes red. The systemic arteries convey the oxygenated (red) blood pumped out by the left ventricle to the cells of the body where it gives off oxygen, takes up carbon dioxide, and becomes blue. The arterial wall has three layers (intima-- inner portion, media -- middle portion, and adventitia -- outer portion).

Atherosclerosis (also known as Hardening of the Arteries or Arteriosclerosis) - *A biochemical arterial disease of epidemic proportions* in developed countries that causes more deaths than all types of cancer, accidents, and infections combined. It is due in large measure to smoking; obtaining too many calories from low-fiber carbohydrates, refined sugar, saturated fats, and *trans* fatty acids; leading a sedentary life; becoming obese from storing large quantities of fat; and letting undue stress control and distort our lives.

This disease causes the inner portion of the arterial wall to become thick, inelastic, and hardened due to plaques formed by infiltration of LDL cholesterol, other fats, and variable amounts of calcium from the blood. Plaques with lots of calcification are hard and those with little are soft and usually small. Many soft plaques develop a central collection (core) of thick, slimy, fatty fluid that is covered over by a thin cap of fibrous tissue. If the cap ruptures, the deadly fluid in the core oozes into the channel where it activates the platelets which causes the blood to clot and close the flow channel (Fig. 34, p. 74). Plaque rupture is the most common cause of heart attacks.

Atherosclerosis often makes the arterial flow surface lose its delicate lining of endothelial cells as the inner wall becomes rough, irregular, and ulcerated. If the blood flow slows or becomes turbulent, the diseased flow surface may activate the platelets and cause clots to form which block the channel and stop the flow of blood (Fig. 35, p. 75). Whether by this process or by rupture of a soft plaque with a lipid core, the flow channel can become blocked by harmful clots which cause heart attacks, strokes, high blood pressure, kidney failure, decreased walking capacity, and amputations. The onset of heart disease occurs about 10 years later in women than men (*p.* 88). Heart attacks and sudden death strike about 20 years later than in men. This delay reflects the earlier protection by estrogens.

In a lesser number of patients, the atherosclerotic process weakens the arterial wall so much, most commonly of the aorta in the abdomen, that the blood pressure forces the wall to bulge out and form enlargements called aneurysms, which may rupture and cause fatal hemorrhage.

There is a current suspicion, as yet insufficiently proven, that the bacterium, *Chlamydia pneumoniae,* as well as some viruses, may infect the arterial wall and be part of the "hardened" artery problem. The question of which comes first, like the chicken or the egg, will be the subject of future research.

Blood Pressure -- Arterial (systemic) - The force that flowing blood exerts against the arterial wall. Two pressures are measured:
  1. S*ystolic pressure*. This is the highest pressure that occurs in the arteries when the heart contracts and pumps blood into the aorta.
  2. D*iastolic pressure*. This is the lowest pressure that occurs in the arteries while the heart is filling before its next beat.

Capillaries - The tiniest blood vessels. Capillary networks connect the smallest arteries to the smallest veins. The capillaries wind between and around the cells to bring them what they must have and remove what they don't need. No cell can be further away from its feeding capillary than the width of the finest hair.

Capillary walls are composed of a single layer of endothelial cells through which oxygen, water, nutrients, and other chemicals diffuse from the blood into all the body's cells, while carbon dioxide and other waste products diffuse from the cells into the blood.

Carbohydrates (plant foods--also *see* Fiber, pp. 283, 284) - Organic compounds constructed of carbon, hydrogen, and oxygen, usually in a ratio of 1:2:1. Most of these compounds are polysaccharides which are called complex carbohydrates. They are broken down in the intestines by the digestive enzymes into $C_6H_{12}O_6$ monosaccharides (simple sugars), *i.e., glucose* and its isomers,* *fructose* (fruit sugar) and *galactose* (from lactose, milk sugar). These monosaccharides are absorbed into the blood. The isomers are converted slowly into glucose by the liver, accounting for their low glycemic indices (p. 284). Glucose is carried by the blood to the cells where, by the action of insulin, it is used to produce energy. *Sucrose* ($C_{12}H_{22}O_{11}$) -- table sugar -- (processed from sugar cane and sugar beets) is a disaccharide which is quickly broken down into glucose and fructose by the addition of water ("hydrolysis"). The cells of the brain and retina can only use glucose for energy; other cells can also use fatty acids for energy.

Excess glucose in plants and animals is stored in the same form $(C_6H_{10}O_5)x$, called starch in plants and *glycogen* in animals. *Insulin,* a hormone secreted by the beta cells of the pancreatic islets in response to increased levels of glucose in the blood, enables the body's cells to use glucose for energy and converts any excess into glycogen, which is stored 1/3 in the liver and 2/3 in muscles. A bit less than a pound of glycogen can be stored in the entire body. Above this level, glucose is rapidly converted into saturated fat and stored in the fat cells of the fatty tissue throughout the body. High levels of insulin block the use of fat for energy. When glucose levels fall due to fasting or exercise, a rise in *glucagon,* a hormone secreted by the alpha cells of the pancreatic islets, converts glycogen back into glucose. When all the glycogen is used, the blood glucose falls and the insulin levels decrease. This allows fat to be used for energy.

Carbon Dioxide (CO_2) - Compound formed in cells when oxygen combines with the carbons of glucose, fat, and protein, and releases energy. Carbon dioxide passes from the cells into the venous blood which carries it to the lungs. In the lungs the carbon dioxide diffuses into the tiny air sacs (the alveoli) where it is exhaled to the outside.

* Isomers - Compounds having the same percentage composition of atoms
  but with different properties due to different arrangement of the atoms.

Cardiac Arrest and Ventricular Fibrillation (Sudden cardiac death) - Cardiac arrest, a state in which the heart suddenly stops beating and remains still. Ventricular fibrillation also means that the heart suddenly stops beating, but it doesn't lie still. Instead, the fibrillating heart at first wiggles vigorously, like a mass of angry angleworms. Then, as the oxygen and nutrient supplies are quickly exhausted, it moves less and less until after a few minutes the heart stops completely and lies motionless in a dilated, flaccid state.

In both conditions, no blood is pumped, and the blood pressure drops abruptly to zero. Unless the circulation can be restored within *four minutes*, the brain cells will be *irreparably damaged* by lack of oxygen. CPR -- Cardiopulmonary Resuscitation -- **must be started before this happens**. Quick action is essential for success(Fig. 99, p. 259). The fibrillating heart must be shocked into standstill with an electric current from a device called a defibrillator before it can start beating again. CPR and drugs to support the myocardium enable many people to recover and live for years.

Cardiologist - A doctor who specializes in the diagnosis and treatment of heart disease. Formerly cardiologists used only measures such as diet, exercise, drugs, and rest to treat patients. Today, many cardiologists also pass catheters -- some with special devices attached to their distal ends (inflatable balloons -- often with stents, cutting instruments, rotating burrs, and ultrasound probes) -- into the coronary arteries and chambers of the heart both for the diagnosis and treatment of disease. In addition, cardiologists often pass leads with electronic components into the right side of the heart for pacemaking and defibrillation purposes.

Cardiopulmonary Resuscitation (CPR) - An emergency measure to maintain life when the heart stops. CPR consists of forcing air into the lungs by mouth-to-mouth respiration (or with a breathing bag if one is available) in a sequence alternating with pushing the lower part of the sternum inward against the front of the heart to restore the circulation. This "breathe and compress" sequence propels the blue blood returning from the body on through the right side of the heart into the lungs where it gains oxygen and loses carbon dioxide. CPR propels this blood, now red, on through the pulmonary veins into the left side of the heart and then on to all the cells of the body (p. 259).

Cerebral Vascular Accident (CVA) - A condition more commonly referred to as a stroke or brain attack. Stroke patients show loss of brain function, such as the inability to move one side of the body, feel, speak, see, comprehend, and many other neurological deficits. Strokes are caused by blockage of the supply of red blood to some part of the brain. This obstruction is generally caused by one of the following three conditions:

1. an *embolus* -- a free-floating fragment of a platelet aggregate, clot, atherosclerotic plaque, or other material which has broken loose from the surface of the inner wall of the heart or artery and is carried by the blood to the brain where it blocks an artery.
2. a blood *clot* forming in an artery of the brain.
3. a brain *hemorrhage*.

Cholesterol - A fat-like substance ($C_{25}H_{47}OH$) used by the body in making the retaining walls of all cells, the male and female sex hormones, and the hormones secreted by the outer part (the cortex) of the adrenal gland which controls vital chemistry of stress, minerals, sugar, and water.

Cholesterol is transported in the blood in three forms, high density lipoprotein cholesterol (HDL), low density lipoprotein cholesterol (LDL), and very low density lipoprotein cholesterol (VLDL). The high concentrations of LDL, low concentrations of HDL, and high levels of triglycerides which are found in VLDL all predispose to the development of atherosclerosis. VLDL and LDL favor atherosclerosis by increasing delivery of cholesterol into the inner portion of the arterial wall. HDL protects against atherosclerosis by transporting LDL to the liver which excretes it in the bile. This lowers the blood level of LDL cholesterol and also removes some from the arterial wall. HDL's high protein content enables it to do this.

Saturated fats and *trans* fatty acids raise LDL cholesterol levels in the blood primarily because they block the receptors for LDL in the liver and in other cells. Excesses of carbohydrates (especially low-fiber types and refined sugar) and proteins also raise LDL levels because they are converted into excess glucose which is processed into saturated fat that blocks more receptors.

In general, LDL cholesterol begins to infiltrate the inner wall of our arteries when the blood level rises above 130 mg/dL. This is the reason why it's so important to: (1) keep our weight under control; and (2) not allow the calories from saturated fats and *trans* fatty acids in our diet to exceed 10% of the total calories we consume in a day. LDL cholesterol is bad only if it gets too high. It's a little like water. We can die of dehydration if we don't have enough, but we can drown in it if we have too much. We need the right amount. LDL cholesterol is the same. Below 100 mg/dL is best.

Collateral Circulation - The blood that flows into the small branches that arise above a blockage and connect with the small vessels that originate below it. The blood flows through these vessels into the main artery below the blockage, and supplies the tissues downstream to whatever extent is possible. These connecting channels are called *collateral vessels* and the blood that flows through them is called *collateral circulation* (Figs. 36, 37; pp. 79, 81).

Common Carotid - From the Greek *karoun,* meaning to stupefy. These vessels were so named by Galen, a Roman physician, in the second century A.D. because compressing them caused loss of consciousness. There is one common carotid artery on each side in the front of the neck. Both arteries extend upward to divide near the angle of the jaw into the internal and external carotid arteries. Each *internal* carotid artery continues upward to pass through an opening in the base of the skull to supply the eye and the front and middle parts of the brain on its side. Each *external* carotid artery continues upward outside the skull to supply the face, mouth, tongue, ear, and scalp on this same side.

Common Femoral Artery - Big artery in each groin that supplies red blood to the entire leg.

Common Iliac Artery - Artery that supplies red blood to half of pelvis and entire leg below, formed by division of abominal aorta at level of navel. There are two of these vessels named, respectively, the right and left common iliac arteries. Both divide into the *internal iliac artery* (which supplies red blood to its half of the pelvis) and the *external iliac artery* (which supplies red blood to the leg below).

Coronary Arteries - Arteries that supply red blood to the heart muscle. There are two of these vessels, a right and a left. They are the first branches of the aorta, and rise from its base. These two arteries and their network of branches spread over the heart like a crown ("corona"), hence their name -- *coronaries*. They enable the right ventricle to pump blue blood to the lungs and the left ventricle to pump red blood to the body.

Coronary Bypass Surgery - Surgery that involves joining grafts that convey arterial (red) blood from an artery outside the heart to the open coronary arteries beyond sites of obstruction in these vessels. This new supply of red blood bypasses the sites of blockage and supplies oxygen, water, nutrients, and other chemicals to the deprived tissues.

Superficial veins (the greater saphenous -- Fig. 29, p. 61 -- most often) taken from the legs are used as coronary artery bypass grafts (CABGs). The upper end of such a graft is joined to an opening made in the body's biggest artery (the ascending aorta) and the lower end to an opening made in a coronary artery beyond the blockage.

Small arteries are also used as CABGs. The most common of these are the two *internal mammary arteries* that run one on each side of the sternum (breastbone) inside the chest. The upper end of a mammary graft is usually left attached to the arm artery from which it arises. The lower end of the graft is joined to an opening made in a coronary artery beyond the obstruction.

Coronary Heart Disease Due to Atherosclerosis - A condition in which there is an insufficient supply of oxygenated (red) blood to the heart muscle because the coronary arteries have become narrowed or even closed off as a result of hardening and thickening of their walls and clot formation on their flow surfaces (coronary thrombosis).

This clotting occurs most often as a consequence of rupture of the lipid core of a soft plaque that releases its fatty contents into the lumen where these "poisonous" lipids activate the platelets and cause the blood to jell, *i.e.,* clot (Fig. 34, p.74). If the artery clots off suddenly, the person may "drop dead." Coronary thrombosis also occurs from platelet aggregation and fibrin formation on rough, irregular, often ulcerated atherosclerotic surfaces that have lost their covering of endothelial cells (Fig. 35, p. 75).

Patients with coronary disease often experience pain in the left side of the front of their chest with exercise or emotion. If you have this symptom (angina), see your doctor promptly.

Diabetes - A condition characterized by thirst, fatigue, high blood sugar, increased output of urine, and decreased ability of the cells to use glucose due to lack of - or insensitivity to - insulin (a hormone secreted by the beta cells of the pancreatic islets). Diabetes, the most common cause of blindness and kidney failure, predisposes to hypertension and atheroslcerosis. Heart disease kills most diabetics.

There are two types of diabetes, type 1 (juvenile) and type 2 (adult onset). Of the 16 million diabetics in the U.S., one million are type 1, and 15 million are type 2. Type 1 diabetes occurs most often around puberty (but can occur in adults). Many researchers believe that this type of diabetes is due to a viral infection which causes lymphocytes of the immune system to destroy the beta cells of the pancreatic islets. When this happens, the pancreas can't make insulin and the individual must then receive daily injections of this hormone for life. But new research suggests that islet transplants *may* help these people.

Type 2 diabetes occurs most frequently in middle-aged, obese adults. But this type is being seen with increasing frequency in younger, obese adults and even in obese children. For unknown reasons, many fat people become resistant to insulin. To compensate, the pancreas secretes more insulin. This works until the exhausted islet cells cannot secrete enough insulin. The initial (and often successful) treatment of type 2 diabetes (about 2200 new cases in the U.S. are diagnosed daily) consists of a diet and exercise program to lose excess fat and add muscle. If such a program isn't adequate, insulin injections and/or oral medications to stimulate the pancreas to secrete more insulin will be necessary. *Prevention is preferable.*

Embolus - An object that has broken loose from the heart or vessel wall -- such as a free-floating fragment of a platelet aggregate, a portion of a clot, or a particle of an atherosclerotic deposit -- and is carried by the blood until it reaches a vessel that is too small to pass through. An arterial embolus plugs the artery at that point and blocks the flow of red blood to the tissues; a venous (pulmonary) embolus goes to the lungs and blocks the flow of blue blood to the alveoli.

Endovascular Surgery - A recent surgical specialty that differs from open vascular surgery in the way the surgeon reaches a diseased vessel. The <u>endovascular</u> surgeon reaches the diseased artery through the flow channel; the <u>vascular</u> surgeon reaches the artery from the outside by cutting through the tissues covering it. For an obstruction, the vascular surgeon opens the artery and removes the blockage or places a bypass graft around it. For an aneurysm, the vascular surgeon incises the wall and places a graft inside the channel.

In endovascular surgery, the surgeon approaches the obstructed artery or aneurysm from the inside, i.e., through the flow channel, with catheters (long, slender, hollow tubes). For an obstruction of the channel, the endovascular surgeon removes the blockage from inside the artery by devices attached to the far end of the catheter (*see* "cardiologist," p. 275). For an aneurysm, the endovascular surgeon places the graft from inside the channel without opening the wall.

The endovascular surgeon passes these catheters over guide wires into the arteries that are to be treated. This new type of surgeon, with the guidance of continuous x-ray visualization, advances guide wires, catheters, operating devices, and grafts into the proper location, often distant, as in the aorta or coronary arteries, and performs the endovascular operation. Endovascular techniques are revolutionizing the surgery of diseased blood vessels. What the future holds cannot be foretold. One thing, however, is certain -- *the impossible of today will become the possible of tomorrow.*

Fats (Triglycerides) - Molecules that consist of three fatty acids chemically linked to a three-carbon chain alcohol called glycerol. All fats contain mixtures of different types of fatty acids. Fatty acids consist of linear chains of carbon atoms with hydrogen atoms bound to them. Ninety-five percent of the fat stored in the fat cells of the adipose tissue is in the triglyceride form. The adipose (fat) cells of the adipose (fatty) tissue have a huge capacity to store fat.

Fats may be classified as saturated or unsaturated. A saturated fatty acid has no double carbon=carbon bonds; all of the bonding sites are filled with hydrogen atoms. Unsaturated fatty acids contain one or more double carbon=carbon bonds. If a fatty acid has only one double bond, it is called monounsaturated. If it has two or more, it is polyunsaturated.

Saturated fats (except for tropical oils such as coconut, palm, and palm kernel types) are solids at room temperature, while unsaturated fats (oils) are liquid. Both varieties are insoluble in water.

The body can make all but two of the many fatty acids it needs. These "essential" acids are the polyunsaturated alpha linolenic and linoleic acids. Because we can't make them, they must be in our diet.

Linoleic acid has a double bond between carbons 6 and 7 (omega-6). Alpha linolenic acid has a double bond between carbons 3 and 4 (omega-3). The ideal ratio of omega-6 to omega-3 fatty acids is about 4:1, or even lower. In the average American's diet, the ratio is much higher, often being an unfavorable 20:1 or worse.

Each fat or oil is a unique combination of saturated, monounsaturated, and polyunsaturated fatty acids. Olive (mainly omega-9 oleic acid), canola, avocado, and peanut oils are primarily monounsaturated and are protective against atherosclerosis. Corn oil (high in omega-6 linoleic acid) is not protective. Salmon, tuna, sardines, trout, mackerel, and flaxseed are especially rich sources of omega-3 alpha linolenic fatty acids which are highly protective against atherosclerosis. Sources of this omega-3 fatty acid, ranked in order of most to least, are shown next in staircase manner:

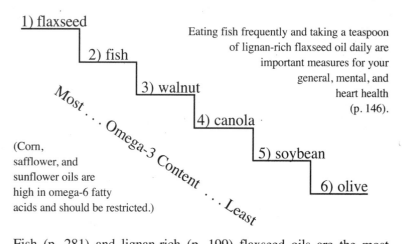

1) flaxseed

2) fish

3) walnut

4) canola

5) soybean

6) olive

Most ... Omega-3 Content ... Least

Eating fish frequently and taking a teaspoon of lignan-rich flaxseed oil daily are important measures for your general, mental, and heart health (p. 146).

(Corn, safflower, and sunflower oils are high in omega-6 fatty acids and should be restricted.)

Fish (p. 281) and lignan-rich (p. 199) flaxseed oils are the most protective against atherosclerosis and harmful clot formation.

Diets high in saturated fats and *trans* fatty acids increase the blood level of LDL cholesterol. This is so because the saturated fats and *trans* fatty acids reduce the activity of the LDL receptors which is the main mechanism whereby LDL cholesterol is removed from the blood stream by the cells of the body, primarily by those in the liver. High LDL cholesterol damages the inner portion of the arterial wall.

Prime sources of saturated fats are fatty meats, unskinned poultry (skin contains nearly all the fat), whole milk, cheeses, butter, cream, ice cream, candies, cakes, pies, and most other desserts.

Prime sources of *trans* fatty acids (pp. 142, 290) are hydrogenated or partially hydrogenated vegetable oils, such as soybean and canola oils, which are used in the manufacture of margarines, especially the hard types, and in many types of cookies, crackers, cakes, candies, chips, dips, doughnuts, pies, and other pastries. Hydrogenation adds hydrogen and converts unsaturated liquid fats (oils) into more saturated solid fats. Beware if the content label reads "hydrogenation" to any degree. ***Recently, however, the FDA has approved two promising new margarines, "Benacol" and "Take Control," that have been treated with plant sterols. These new margarines have been shown to lower LDL cholesterol by 10-15%.***

Phospholipids, fats that contain phosphorus, are essential building materials for the walls of the 100 trillion cells that make up our bodies. If these membranes were to dissolve in water, we would die in seconds. Their fat content prevents this. In addition, our brain is 60% fat. The right fats, such as monounsaturated omega-9 olive and polyunsaturated omega-3 fish and flaxseed oils, are needed by the cells. But, we must restrict saturated fats and *trans* fatty acids because they damage the inner walls of our arteries (p. 282).

Protective (unsaturated) fats (*see* above and pp. 281, 282) are not only good for us, they add taste and satisfaction to our meals. But they are such a rich source of calories (9 calories/gram) that they must be eaten in moderation to maintain balance in our diet. If we don't eat for 12 to 18 hours or run for many miles, our main source of energy shifts from glucose to fatty acids as our meager stores of glycogen (storage form of glucose) are quickly used up (p. 274).

Fiber - (*also see* Carbohydrates, p. 274) The portion of plant foods that our bodies can't digest. There are two basic types of fiber: soluble and insoluble. Insoluble fiber helps the digestive system run smoothly and prevents constipation. This fiber, referred to as "roughage," includes the woody parts of plants, such as the skins of fruits and vegetables and the outer coating of grain and rice kernels.

Soluble fiber dissolves and thickens in water to form gels. Beans, barley, broccoli, citrus fruits, oatmeal, and especially oat bran are rich sources of soluble fiber. This type of fiber decreases the absorption of cholesterol by the small intestines.

Fiber is found only in complex carbs. Whether the fiber is soluble or insoluble, complex carbs that are coated by their natural protective fiber components are digested and absorbed more slowly than when the fiber has been removed by refining processes. A high-fiber content slows the digestion of complex carbs and decreases the glucose load on the pancreas. This lowers the secretion of insulin and reduces the risk of developing type 2 diabetes (pp. 279, 280).

This is why the majority of our carbohydrate calories should come from high-fiber sources, such as fresh fruits; fresh vegetables; and legumes (peas, beans, and lentils); whole-grain breads, cereals, and pastas; and whole grains, such as brown rice. **The Better Life Diet** is high-fiber. It is designed to prevent heart disease and type 2 diabetes.

This is also why we should markedly restrict the calories we get from low-fiber, processed, complex carbohydrates (such as white bread, mashed potatoes, french fries -- also have too much fat -- and white rice) because they have lost most of their protective fiber and are rapidly digested into glucose. Refined sugar (mainly sucrose), a totally non-fiber, disaccharide carbohydrate, $(C_{12}H_{22}O_{11})$, combines with water in the intestines and is quickly converted into glucose and its isomer, fructose, which are both $C_6H_{12}O_6$ monosaccharides. Because excess glucose can be seriously dangerous over time to our health, we should drastically restrict low-fiber carbs and refined sugar in our diet (pp. 138, 279, 280, 289, 290).

Fiber is also valuable because it contains many minerals, phytochemicals (plant chemicals), and vitamins.

Glycemic Index - Ranks a carbohydrate food on how high it raises the blood glucose in comparison to the elevation caused by ingesting pure glucose. The lower a food's index, the less that food raises the blood glucose.

Heart Attack - A condition in which part of the heart wall dies because of lack of blood supply, most often from obstruction (occlusion) of a coronary artery due to atherosclerosis and clot formation (thrombosis). The impact of a heart attack may be mild, moderate, severe, or even fatal depending on how much and which part of the heart muscle has lost its blood supply. The patient suffering a heart attack will often experience severe chest pain, become nauseated, sweat profusely, develop marked shortness of breath, have low blood pressure, and feel very weak.

Hemoglobin - The iron containing protein in the red cells of our blood which combines with oxygen in the lungs to form a bright red compound called *oxyhemoglobin*. The red blood cells carry the oxyhemoglobin to the tissues where it supplies oxygen to the cells so they can live. After giving up oxygen, hemoglobin becomes a dark burgundy color and is called *reduced hemoglobin*. The more oxygen the blood gives up, the darker (more blackish) it becomes.

The change in color of hemoglobin in the pulmonary capillaries causes the blood in the pulmonary veins and systemic arteries to be bright red, and the change in the color of hemoglobin in the systemic capillaries causes the blood in our systemic veins and pulmonary arteries to be dark burgundy in color. Though not strictly accurate, venous blood is referred to as "blue."

Hemorrhage (Bleeding) - Loss of blood from a blood vessel. In external hemorrhage, the blood escapes from the body. In internal hemorrhage, the bleeding occurs into a body cavity or into the tissues surrounding the bleeding vessel.

High Blood Pressure (Hypertension) - Persistent or intermittent elevation of blood pressure above upper range of normal - 140/90 (130/80 for diabetics). Uncontrolled, chronic high blood pressure strains the heart; damages arteries; and creates a greater risk of heart attack, sudden cardiac death, congestive heart failure, stroke, kidney failure, blindness, and hemorrhage from aneurysm rupture.

Infarct - An area of tissue that has died as a result of lack of blood supply. A "myocardial infarct" is an area of dead heart muscle due to the blockage of its blood flow by obstruction of the coronary artery which supplied it.

Insulin - A hormone secreted by the beta cells of the islets of the pancreas in response to the level of glucose in the blood. The higher the glucose, the more insulin the beta cells secrete. Insulin enables all the cells of the body to use glucose for energy, converts extra glucose into glycogen for storage in the liver and muscles, and stops the use of fat for energy (pp. 35,144,279,280). When the glycogen stores are filled, insulin converts any excess blood glucose into saturated fat which is stored in the cells of the adipose tissue.

Intermittent Claudication - "Claudication," Latin for "lameness." Painful state brought on by exercise and relieved by rest. The most common cause of this condition is the obstructive form of atherosclerosis that prevents delivery of an adequate supply of red blood to the contracting muscles.The calf muscles are most frequently affected. The more restricted the blood supply, the shorter the distance a person can walk before cramping pain forces him/her to stop and rest the aching muscles. The muscle pain that develops during exercise is due to a progressively increasing accumulation of lactic acid in and around the blood-deprived, contracting muscle cells. During the pain-imposed rest periods, the blood supply "catches up" and removes the lactic acid. The pain disappears as this happens.

Ischemia - A condition in which there is either an insufficient supply of arterial (red) blood to a part of the body due to obstruction of the artery supplying it and/or a reduced output of blood by the heart.

Life Style - An individual's typical way of life, including home environment, diet, occupation, recreational pursuits, exercise routines, and smoking, drinking, and sleeping habits.

Lumen (channel) - The passageway inside a tubular organ. The lumen is the channel for blood to flow inside a blood vessel.

Metabolism - A general term designating all chemical changes that occur in the body.

Murmur - The sound generated by blood swirling within the heart or arteries. This turbulence (swirling) occurs in the blood as it jets suddenly from a narrow channel into a large one.

Obesity - A condition characterized by distension of the adipocytes (fat cells) of the adipose (fatty) tissue from storage of excess fat in them, which predisposes the obese person to type 2 diabetes (p. 279,280), blindness, kidney failure, hypertension, atherosclerosis, clots, heart attacks, sudden death, congestive heart failure, strokes, limb loss, cancer, gallstones, and degenerative arthritis. Fat accumulations in and around the abdomen (central obesity-apple shape) are most dangerous.

Occlusion of a Blood Vessel - The closing or shutting off of a blood vessel's lumen (flow channel).

Open-Heart Surgery - Surgery performed on the opened heart under direct vision.

Osteoporosis - A condition that depletes bone structure, shortens stature, weakens the skeleton, and causes fractures, especially of the hips, spine, ribs, and wrists to occur in the advancing years of one of every two women and one of eight men over age 50.

Peripheral Vascular Disease - A term which, in its broadest sense, refers to diseases of any of the blood vessels outside of the heart and to diseases of the lymph vessels.

Plaque - An area of scar tissue and necrosis in the inner portion of the wall of an artery caused by infiltration of LDL cholesterol and other fats. The plaque may be hard if much calcium is deposited in or around it, or soft if little is deposited. Small, soft plaques often develop a lipid core which can rupture and cause the blood to clot (pp. 272, 273). This is the most common cause of heart attacks.

Plasma - The cell-free liquid portion of uncoagulated blood; serum is the liquid that remains after blood clots.

Platelets - Tiny pinched off parts of a large cell in the bone marrow called a megakaryocyte. These fragments, called "platelets," survive about 10 days after they are released into the blood from the bone marrow. Each second, about 1.5 million wear out and are replaced by 1.5 million new ones. Too few platelets can cause us to bleed to death; too many can cause us to clot to death.

Platelets, being very light, float along in the outer portion of the blood stream ever ready to be activated. When activated by an injury, they can initiate formation of beneficial clots to plug holes in the wall. In addition, platelets contain many growth factors that promote the healing of wounds. Regrettably, platelets can also be activated by the athersclerotic arterial wall to form harmful clots (Figs. 34,35; pp. 74,75).

Proteins - Complex, big molecules constructed of long, three-dimensionally wrapped chains of combinations of amino acids. Amino acids are molecules constructed of four chemical units joined to a single carbon atom: an amino (NH_2) group, a hydrogen atom (H), a carboxylic acid (COOH) group, and a side-group containing various combinations of carbon, hydrogen, nitrogen (N), and sometimes sulfur (S). It is the side-groups that distinguish the 20 different amino acids that our bodies must have. Of these amino acids, nine can't be manufactured by our bodies and must be derived from the foods we eat. These amino acids, which we must have but can't manufacture, are called *essential* amino acids.

The body manufactures thousands of different types of proteins from different combinations of these 20 amino acids. Each of these proteins has a single function, such as that of an enzyme, which is determined by the order and shape of its amino acid chains.

Many vital structures inside our cells are made from proteins. For example, the ribosomes that make proteins, and the mitochondria that make energy are constructed with proteins. The enzymes controlling the chemistry of our bodies are proteins. The hemoglobin in our red blood cells carrying vital oxygen is a protein. Our muscles are proteins. The external surface features of our bodies (eyes, ears, nose, skin, hair, and nails) are made of proteins.

As discussed previously, obesity can lead to many serious medical problems. On the other hand, being very thin is also very dangerous. If people who are very thin become unable to eat for some reason, their depleted muscles are progressively consumed for energy since they have no glycogen or fat stores to sustain them. Under these conditions, muscle tissue is converted into glucose by a process called "gluconeogenesis." In chronic starvation, death occurs when the body has consumed about half its muscle tissue for energy. Clearly, proteins are essential for life. Also, they provide taste and satisfaction to our meals. Proteins are best obtained from fish, skinless poultry, eggs, peas, beans, lentils, nuts, seeds, nonfat/low-fat dairy products, low-fat meat, such as lean beef, lamb, and center-cut pork loin/chop or roast, and shellfish (p. 138).

Pulse - The expansion of an artery which can be palpated with a finger when the heart contracts (systole) and pumps blood out into the aorta and its branches.

Risk Factors - Conditions that predispose to the development of a certain disease. Risk factors for having a heart attack include:
- Smoking.
- Eating a diet high in low-fiber carbohydrates, refined sugar, saturated fats, *trans* fatty acids, and calories.
- Leading a sedentary life.
- Carrying significant excess weight (fat).
- Experiencing marked stress.
- Having a family history of heart disease.
- Possessing sticky platelets; low blood levels of HDL cholesterol and omega-3 fatty acids; and high blood levels of fibrinogen, LDL cholesterol, triglycerides, homocysteine, and/or blood sugar.
- Suffering from high blood pressure, diabetes, gout, and/or low thyroid function.

Saphenous Vein - The greater saphenous vein, the longest vein in the body, runs just beneath the skin along the inside of the leg from ankle to groin where it then goes deep to join the big vein (the common femoral) at that level. The patient's own saphenous veins are the most frequently used grafts to bypass obstructions of the coronary arteries of the heart and the arteries of the leg.

Sclerosis - A thickening or hardening of a body part, as in the term "atherosclerosis," indicates that the arterial wall has became hard.

Stress - (Please *see* p. 188)

Sugar, Refined (Sucrose, $C_{12}H_{22}O_{11}$, p. 274) - a non-fiber dissacharide (carbohydrate) with a sweet taste that is refined in crystalline or powdered form from sugar cane or sugar beets for use in foods to improve taste. Table sugar has only calories -- no fiber, minerals, phytochemicals (plant chemicals), or vitamins. Sucrose is quickly combined with water in the intestines and converted into glucose and its isomer, fructose, which are both $C_6H_{12}O_6$

monosaccharides. This hydrolytic reaction occurs at least as fast as the digestion of low-fiber carbs (pp. 274,283,284). Thus, we should drastically restrict refined sugar and low-fiber carbs in our diet. They both yield glucose which stimulates insulin secretion. Insulin converts surplus glucose into fat and prevents its use for energy. If allowed to persist, *glucose excess* will cause obesity and, frequently, type 2 diabetes (pp. 279, 280) with its many complications of blindness, kidney failure, hypertension, atherosclerosis, clots, heart attacks, sudden death, congestive heart failure, strokes, decreased walking capacity, limb loss, gallstones, and degenerative arthritis.

Syndrome X - Condition affecting a growing number of people identified by the chemical triad of low HDL cholesterol, high triglycerides, and a decreased sensitivity to high blood levels of insulin. This triad is associated with a strong tendency to develop central (abdominal) obesity, type 2 diabetes, hypertension, and atherosclerosis with its many complications. The **Better Life Diet and Exercise Program** is well-suited to treat this disorder.

Trans **Fatty Acids** (Fats, pp. 281-283) - an altered form of vegetable oils produced by the process of hydrogenation which adds hydrogen atoms to the unsaturated carbon chains which converts these liquid oils into soft solids at room temperature. These hydrogenated chains resemble those of saturated fats and are called *trans* fatty acids. Examples of such changes are found in the conversion of soybean and canola oils into soft solids in the manufacture of margarines, and of peanut oil in the manufacture of peanut butter. These altered oils are as dangerous to your heart as saturated fats, both blocking the LDL receptors in the liver (p. 282).

Veins - Vessels that carry blood back to the heart. The systemic veins convey the deoxygenated (blue) blood from the body to the right side of the heart. The pulmonary veins convey the freshly oxygenated (red) blood from the lungs to the left side of the heart. Though veins have much thinner walls than arteries, they have the same layers: intima, media, and adventitia (Figs. 26,28; pp. 57,60).

Vitamins - Organic compounds vital for our growth and function which we can't make and, therefore, must have in our diets.

Review Questions
(Answers found on pages as listed)

1. If you were God, how would you build the human body? **1-316.**

2. What is the boundary organ concept? **40-43**

3. What are the three main parts of the cardiovascular system? **20, 45, 56, 64**

4. What makes the blood in systemic arteries red and the blood in systemic veins blue? **46,47,284,285**

5. What do platelets and fibrinogen have to do with blood clotting? **67-71**

6. Are "hardening of the arteries" and "atherosclerosis" the same thing? **4,72**

7. Is it true that hardening of the arteries and clot formation kill more people in the United States than cancer, accidents, and infections combined? **5**

8. What are the two main complications of atherosclerosis? **77-79,82,83**

9. Where do arterial blockages occur most commonly? **87**

10. Where do aneurysms develop most often? **82,108,109**

11. What is "angina"? **90**

12. What are hard and soft plaques? **73-75**

13. What is a "heart attack"? **89,284**

14. What is the most common cause of heart attacks? **73-75, 272,273**

15. What are the lifestyle risk factors associated with the development of atherosclerosis and clot formation? **115**

16. What are the signs of a heart attack (**88,89**), a TIA (**98**), a stroke (**94,95**), a kidney that lacks an adequate blood supply (**102,103**), and a leg that doesn't have enough blood supply (**104-107**)?

17. How are aneurysms diagnosed? **108-111**

18. How can 90% of premature deaths from cardiovascular disease be prevented? **112-249, 254-266**

19. Why do long-term, heavy smokers die an average of six to eight years sooner than nonsmokers? **115-118,120**

20. What is a "carbohydrate," a "fat," and a "protein"? **274,281-283, 288**

21. What is the difference between HDL cholesterol and LDL cholesterol? **73**

22. Why should saturated fats and *trans* fatty acids be severely restricted? **140,142,276,277,281-283,289,290**

23. Why should low-fiber carbohydrates and refined sugar be severely restricted? **115,137,138,140,143,283,284**

24. What is "fiber"? **283,284**

25. Why are high-fiber carbohydrates good for you but low-fiber carbohydrates are not? **138,139,144,283,284**

26. What is the "glycemic index"? **284**

27. Why are high glycemic index foods bad, and low glycemic foods good for you? **138,139,144,283,284**

28. Where does 90% of the salt in our diet come from? **199**

29. What is insulin? **35,285**

30. What is diabetes? **279,280**

31. What are type 1 and type 2 diabetes? **279,280**

32. How does insulin cause obesity? **144,150,285**

33. How does obesity cause type 2 diabetes? **279,280,286,287**

34. What are the complications of diabetes? **279,280,290**

35. How does a diet high in low-fiber, complex carbohydrates and refined sugar cause diabetes? **138,139,143-145,279,280,283,284**

36. What's wrong with the "Standard American Diet"? **137**

37. What are the seven guidelines of the **Better Life Diet**? **138,139**

38. Who should follow the **Better Life Diet**? **141**

39. What is "Syndrome X"? **290**

40. What must one do to successfully lose excess fat, add muscle, and then maintain that desired weight? **150-152**

41. Why is aerobic exercise essential for health? **115, 161-163**

42. Is the simple "talk test" all you need to find the aerobic exercise pace that's right for you? **161-165**

43. What makes walking such a good exercise for nearly everyone? **174,175**

44. What are the five cardinal rules and three additional strategies for heart-healthy living? **190-199**

45. What do the letters -- S ... D E W ... S -- help you remember? **192-194**

46. What are the two general types of operations for arterial disease? **202**

47. How is endovascular surgery performed? **206-211**

48. What is a "CABG"? **213,218-223,278**

49. What is a "PTCA"? **208-211**

50. What is an endovascular stent and how does it work? **208,209,211**

51. How does an artificial pacemaker for the heart work? **254-257**

52. How should "CPR" be performed? **258-260**

53. Whom do you call when a heart emergency occurs, and what information do you give? **258-260**

54. What is an "AICD"? **261-263**

55. Why were there only 2,500 heart transplants done in the United States last year? **264**

56. Are there reliable guidelines to help you find increased happiness in life? **267-270**

About the Author

LESTER R. SAUVAGE, MD, graduate of the St. Louis University School of Medicine at age 21 in 1948, author and world-renowned heart surgeon and research scientist, is clinical professor of surgery emeritus at the University of Washington and Founder of The Hope Heart Institute in Seattle where he is also Medical Director Emeritus. He has authored 252 articles on heart and blood vessel research and surgery, a monograph on heart valve replacement, an acclaimed inspirational book, *The Open Heart: Secret to Happiness,* and *The Better Life Diet,* in addition to this volume, *You Can Beat Heart Disease,* Moreover, he pioneered the first experimental coronary bypass surgery using veins and the first use of the internal thoracic arteries to revascularize the entire human heart. Also, he pioneered the development of a line of artifical arteries, known as the *Sauvage Graft,* that have been used world-wide.

Dr. Sauvage is certified by the American Board of Surgery and the American Board of Thoracic Surgery. He has also been awarded certificates for special competence in the surgery of infants and children and in vascular surgery by the American Board of Surgery.

His many honors and awards include:
- Member, Alpha Omega Alpha National Honorary Medical Society, 1947.
- Member, Alpha Sigma Nu National Jesuit Honor Society, 1948.
- The degree HONORIS CAUSA, Seattle University, 1976.
- The Brotherhood Award, National Conference of
  Christians and Jews, 1979.
- The Clemson Award, Clemson University, for outstanding contributions
  in applied research on biomaterials, 1982.
- The degree of Doctor of Science, Gonzaga University, 1982.
- The Jefferson Award, American Institute for Public Service, 1983.
- The Governor's (Washington State) Distinguished
  Volunteer Award, 1983.
- The Washington State Medal of Merit, 1987.
- Honorary member of the New England Vascular Society, 1987.
- Seattle First Citizen Award, Seattle-King County
  Association of Realtors, 1992.
- Member, The American Surgical Association, 1995.
- Knight, The Equestrian Order of the Holy Sepulchre of Jerusalem, 1995.

About the Prevention Consultant

CAROL P. GARZONA, former Director of Health Communications at The Hope Heart Institute and Editor of the **Hope Health Letter** and related products, received her undergraduate and graduate training in health communication theory and public health at the University of Washington. Carol's publications for the lay public are read by millions of people each month.

About the Illustration Team

KATHRYN D. BARKER, Medical Artist and Calligrapher, received her undergraduate and graduate degrees in art from the University of Michigan. Kathryn has been actively working in the field of medical art for 20 years and is widely known for the beauty, clarity, and accuracy of her illustrations.

WARREN A. BERRY received his undergraduate training in multimedia production at the University of Washington and subsequently worked for many years at the School of Medicine in CCTV and later in commercial TV before coming to The Hope Heart Institute as Director of Computer Graphics and Medical Photography. His talent and drive have inspired each of us to "get our job done right."

A message from Better Life Press

If you would like
Dr. Sauvage
to speak to your group on subjects such as:

- **Dieting -- pleasure, not punishment.**

- **Five cardinal rules for optimal health.**

- **Surgery should have only a limited role.**

- **National campaign for health and fitness**

- **How to find greater happiness**
  in our extended years.

Call Stan Emert at 206/323-0116, or through the website at **http://www.drsauvage.com**. Dr. Sauvage has spoken to many associations, conventions, schools, business meetings, book clubs, and gatherings of other kinds. Dr. Sauvage accepts a limited number of speaking engagements each year to discuss hope, health and happiness, or, as he says, "The **How** and the **Why** to Live."

For questions concerning bulk purchases of this book, *The Better Life Diet*, or *The Open Heart*, please contact **Better Life Press** at 1210 22nd Ave E, Seattle, Washington, U.S.A. 98112.
Phone: 206/323-0116; http://www.drsauvage.com
E-mail: lsauvage@hopeheart.org

If you are a book retailer or other book seller, please contact **Independent Publishers Group**, 814 N. Franklin Street, Chicago, Illinois, U.S.A. 60610. Phone: 800/888-4741 or 312/337-0747.

Need for Research

When I founded **The Hope Heart Institute** in 1959 there was a pressing need to develop better operations and means with which to treat patients afflicted with heart and blood vessel diseases. During the next 25 years the Institute developed an international reputation as my staff and I made important discoveries, including development of:

1. The coronary bypass operation using veins in 1962.
2. Improved artificial grafts to replace or bypass diseased arteries during the 1970s.
3. Operations to bring blood to the *entire* heart using *only* the internal mammary arteries in 1984.

In the 1980s the Institute broadened its research scope to include prevention as well as treatment of heart disease. These new studies proved successful and pointed the way for future work designed to decrease the need for surgery.

During this same period the Institute developed a major educational mission for the lay public through creation of the **Hope Health Letter**, a monthly publication designed to help healthy people stay healthy. Millions read each issue and millions more read other materials written by the staff.

The 1990s past and 2000s present have been continuous times of expanding investigative excitement at the Institute as its dedicated scientific staff has identified key research questions facing the field of cardiovascular disease and has accepted the challenge of contributing to their solutions. To aid in this effort, departments of Molecular Biology, Vascular Biology, Medical Engineering, and Clinical Research have been added to those established in earlier years -- Chemistry and Hematology, Surgery, Cell Biology, and Vascular Healing.

The discovery by the Institute's staff in the early 1990s that there is a healing cell in the blood which can convert the inner surface of an artificial blood vessel graft into a living natural structure is of the utmost importance. The Institute's staff proved in the mid 1990s that this cell originates in the bone marrow. The Institute is committed in the new millenium to determining how to control this cell's actions for the benefit of humankind.

Such basic scientific information could be of enormous biologic importance because it would:

1. Advance understanding of how blood cells form and blood vessels develop and heal.
2. Direct how to design better artificial blood vessels.
3. Identify ways to deploy this healing cell to rapidly heal such grafts in the coronary arteries of the heart and in the small arteries below the knees.
4. Add knowledge to help prevent hardening of the arteries (the cause of 95% of heart disease).
5. Enable new blood vessels to be formed (angiogenesis) to supply blood to areas lacking adequate supply.
6. Provide new insights as to how to stop tumors from developing the blood supply they need to grow, spread, and kill their victims.

The possibilities for these major advances are real and must be pursued with full intensity because more people still die of heart and artery diseases due to atherosclerosis and clot formation than die of cancer, accidents, and infections combined.

The Hope Heart Institute faces the future with optimism based on past discoveries, current research, and on a passionate belief that these diseases can be defeated in our time.

Though we are still far from victory in this all-out struggle for humankind, I believe that heart and artery diseases as we know them today can be overcome in our time. I see this book as a major force to empower people to help themselves and in turn to help others in this crucial struggle to defeat the Western world's greatest killers, hardening of the arteries (atherosclerosis), and clot formation.

My goal in writing this book has been to help people live longer, healthier, and happier lives. You, the reader, have a vital role to play. I now ask you to take my recommendations from these pages and turn them into your everyday actions. Please encourage your family and friends to do the same. **By working together, I am confident that we will defeat heart disease in our time.**

To join the Hope Heart team, please contact:

The Hope Heart Institute
528 18th Avenue
Seattle, WA 98122
Phone: (206) 903-2254
Fax: (206) 903-2244
www.hopeheart.org

The Institute has outgrown its current facilities and space and must expand, which is expected to cost $20 million. Your kind assistance would further the goal of eradicating heart disease. If you feel as I do, please help, if possible, by sending your tax-exempt gift labeled "Expansion Fund" to the above address.

Thank you,
Lester R. Sauvage, MD

Endorsements

(Continued from front of book)

"I am enthusiastic about this book! Dr. Sauvage has done a remarkable job of condensing an immense amount of anatomy, physiology, pathology, surgery, medicine, nutrition, and psychology -- and even a touch of ethics -- into such a small and easily read volume. It is replete with illustrations that are lucid and to the point.

"This book could serve as an excellent source of good information for any layman interested in cardiovascular disease. More importantly, it is exactly what patients need to help them understand what their doctors tell them. This book will be of *inestimable value* to great numbers of patients whose doctors don't have the time to get their well-intentioned but often inadequate explanations across to them. *You Can Beat Heart Disease* will go a long way to help patients overcome fear and become successful, active, informed participants in their own care.

"I am pleased to give this book *my highest recommendation."*

- **Wiley F. Barker, MD**
Professor of Surgery Emeritus
Division of Vascular Surgery
UCLA School of Medicine, Los Angeles, California

"An *excellent book* for patients and their families. After reading it, I gave my copy to my parents so they could better understand atherosclerosis and how to prevent its impact on their health as they age."

- **Julie Ann Freischlag, MD**
Professor of Surgery
Chief, Division of Vascular Surgery
Director of Vascular Center
UCLA School of Medicine and Medical Center
Los Angeles, California

"This book will *help you* beat heart disease."

> - **John W. Kirklin, MD**
> Professor of Surgery, Department of Surgery
> University of Alabama at Birmingham

"This book is about much more than heart disease, it is a *prescription for good health*, and describes in clear terms how to use this knowledge."

> - **Malcolm O. Perry, MD**
> Chairman of Surgery, St. Paul Medical Center, Dallas, Texas

"Maimonides, 1135-1204, believed that study of the marvels of the human body deepened one's faith in God. He further believed that the acquisition of medical skill and wisdom expanded one's intellectual capacity to recognize the awesome power of human and divine spirituality.

"Dr. Lester Sauvage has achieved all this and more in his very personal presentation of the human body with particular emphasis on the circulatory system. I enjoyed reading this book for many reasons and learned much from it that is ordinarily not appreciated. For example, I never realized how many and how fast red blood cells are recycled! This is a *terrific, easily readable book* that should be required reading by the general public."

> - **Herbert Dardik, MD**
> Clinical Professor of Surgery, Mount Sinai School of Medicine,
> New York, New York
> Chief of Vascular Surgery, Englewood Hospital and Medical Center,
> Englewood, New Jersey

"This book by Dr. Sauvage and his staff focuses clearly on cardiovascular disease, the number one killer of Americans, and emphasizes what we *need to know* about its detection, management, and prevention. Those who carefully read *You Can Beat Heart Disease* will make the lifestyle choices necessary to keep themselves healthy. Just imagine the positive impact on our health care system if we would all do this."

> - **Ronald J. Stoney, MD**
> Professor of Surgery Emeritus
> University of California, San Francisco

"You Can Beat Heart Disease is succinct, highly readable, and authoritative. It should be *invaluable* to readers interested in the primary or secondary prevention of heart disease. Anyone with atherosclerosis will find this well organized text to be very useful, especially should they be considering a revascularization procedure, because well informed patients tend to have markedly better outcomes."

- Floyd D. Loop, MD
Chief Executive Officer
The Cleveland Clinic Foundation, Cleveland, Ohio

"You Can Beat Heart Disease is an excellent overview of the cardiovascular system in language which both interests and informs and is *extremely readable.* The philosophy which Dr. Sauvage promotes is not only sensible and practical but properly emphasizes how our bodies can be made healthier and kept that way, and he rightly stresses the importance of our inner spiritual needs. The book deserves to be widely accepted, and it should be compulsory reading for all medical, nursing, and related professionals."

- S. A. Mellick, CBE, MD
Vascular Surgeon, Brisbane, Australia
Past President (1991-93), International Society for Cardiovascular Surgery

"This outstanding book provides the *essential knowledge* we need to prevent and treat diseases of the heart and arteries. Dr. Sauvage communicates his powerful message in the same passionate manner that he taught me vascular surgery almost thirty years ago."

- Yasutsugu Nakagawa, MD
Director, Division of Cardiovascular Surgery
Chiba Cardiopulmonary Center, Chiba, Japan

"The authors have been able to put the most current information regarding the prevention and treatment of heart disease into proper perspective. This precise, easy-to-read, concise book with fast moving text and beautiful illustrations will dispel confusion and settle controversies for its fortunate readers. In the true sense of the word, this is a *self-help book for everyone."*

- Malay Patel, MD
Vascular Surgeon, Ahmedabad, India

"This remarkable, small volume represents a *precious distillate* of Lester Sauvage's life-long experience with every aspect of the prevention and treatment of diseases of the heart and arteries. Importantly, this concisely written, well illustrated, and easily understood book is potentially a life saving aid for all of us and should be read by everyone."

- **Mr. Aires A.B. Barros D'Sa, MD**
Consultant Vascular Surgeon, Vascular Surgery Unit
Royal Victoria Hospital/The Queen's University, Belfast, United Kingdom

"Here is a collection of valuable, *clearly presented,* in-depth discussions about the causes, prevention, and treatment -- both medical and surgical -- of heart and artery diseases. Preventive measures are stressed, and the spiritual dimensions of life and service to others are unblushingly set out in this concise handbook."

- **C. Rollins Hanlon, MD, FACS**
Executive Consultant, Director General Emeritus
American College of Surgeons, Chicago, Illinois

"This highly readable, up-to-date description of heart and blood vessel problems and their management is a *great book* for professionals and non-professionals alike."

- **Robert L. Kistner, MD**
Straub Clinic & Hospital, Honolulu, Hawaii

"I *enjoyed* reading *this book immensely,* and I firmly believe that an understanding of the physical and spiritual principles underlying the function of the body is essential for a healthy heart."

- **Glenn C. Hunter, MD**
Professor of Surgery, Section of Vascular Surgery
University of Texas Medical Branch, Galveston, Texas

"Lester Sauvage has brought us an invaluable compendium of heart information in a manner we can all understand. This book is a *must for all -- sick or well."*

- **Lloyd M. Nyhus, MD**
Professor of Surgery Emeritus
University of Illinois, Chicago

"You Can Beat Heart Disease is a unique book with the clear objective of helping to defeat heart disease by empowering the reader with easily understandable and highly useful information. This book has been written specifically for the lay public and is *exceptionally well organized.* It begins with an overview of relevant biologic processes, progresses to specific clinical diseases, and then factually discusses the advantages and disadvantages of the prevention and treatment options that are available. Because this book has the information I want my patients and their families to have, I will strongly recommend it to them."

- Howard P. Greisler, MD
Professor of Surgery
Division of Vascular Surgery
Loyola University Medical Center, Maywood, Illinois

"I found Lester Sauvage's new book, *You Can Beat Heart Disease,* to be extremely informative and highly useful -- likely the *best in its class.* I will order it to be distributed to my patients."

- Francis Robicsek, MD, PhD
Chairman, Department of Thoracic and Cardiovascular Surgery
Carolinas Medical Center, Charlotte, North Carolina
Clinical Professor of Surgery, University of North Carolina

"In *You Can Beat Heart Disease,* Dr. Lester Sauvage has provided an invaluable source of information to enlighten the layman about cardiovascular diseases. Beyond the informative and educational sections of this book that will *appeal to all individuals,* including medical personnel, Dr. Sauvage has provided a *practical, common-sense approach to preventive measures.* Additionally, he has provided valuable spiritual insight to help us contend with cardiovascular diseases. In my view, the goal of this book is to help us all live longer, happier, and healthier lives. Clearly, this goal has been accomplished."

- Calvin B. Ernst, MD
Professor of Surgery,
Chief, Division of Vascular Surgery
Allegheny University of the Health Sciences
Philadelphia, Pennsylvania

"Pleasantly informative, scientifically accurate, well illustrated, and *written in grand style.*"

- John J. Bergan, MD
Professor of Surgery
Loma Linda University, Loma Linda, California
University of California, San Diego, California
Uniformed Services University of the Health Sciences, Bethesda, Maryland

"This book was *easy to read* and *easy to understand.* In my opinion, it is an *ideal book* about a *vital subject* that will, I am sure, benefit the general public, cardiovascular patients, and even their doctors."

- Charles G. Rob, MD
Professor of Surgery
Uniformed Services University of the Health Sciences, Bethesda, Maryland
Past President (1959-61), International Society for Cardiovascular Surgery

"I have just finished your book, and I think it is *outstanding.* Congratulations! I hope it becomes a best seller.

"I particularly enjoyed the parts on smoking cessation, dietary management, exercise, and the control of stress. It really *covers all the topics extremely well and is very easy reading and enjoyable.* You have my total support for achieving maximal circulation of this important book. It will help many people, and I will use it for my patients."

- Frank J. Veith, MD
Professor & Chief of Vascular Surgical Services
Montefiore Medical Center &
Albert Einstein College of Medicine
New York, New York

"I read every page of this compact volume and found it to be *most informative.* I predict that it will be very helpful to lay individuals -- and to doctors as well!"

- Jesse E. Thompson, MD, FACS
Vascular Surgeon and Director Emeritus, Division of Vascular Surgery
Baylor University Medical Center, Dallas, Texas
Past President (1983-85), International Society for Cardiovascular Surgery

"This is a *much-needed book* to help the public understand cardiovascular disease, the number one killer in the United States. The book contains up-to-date and easy-to-read information about the mechanisms of the disease processes, the diagnosis, and, most importantly, a clear explanation of the modern treatments for cardiovascular disorders."

- James S.T. Yao, MD, PhD
Magerstadt Professor of Surgery
Northwestern University Medical School, Chicago, Illinois

"Dr. Lester Sauvage and his team have succeeded in the *monumental task* of summarizing the great mound of information relating to atherosclerotic heart and artery disease into a relatively small volume of easily understood English prose suitable for reading by the lay public. My congratulations to them for undertaking this great and worthy task."

- Anthony M. Imparato, MD
Professor of Surgery
Division of Vascular Surgery
New York University Medical Center, New York, New York

This book presents a *clear and concise* overview of cardiovascular disease: its causes, effects, treatment, and prevention. Written in a very readable format with good illustrations, this book will be very useful for patients and their families. It will also be valuable for those of us who wish to avoid the disastrous consequences of hardening of our arteries and clot formation."

- Christopher K. Zarins, MD
Chidester Professor of Surgery and Chief of Vascular Surgery,
Stanford University, Stanford, California

"Dr. Sauvage has had great experience in the surgical management of patients with heart disease. And he has now produced a book, *You Can Beat Heart Disease,* which, if followed, will clearly *reduce the need for heart surgery.* This book will be of particular value to those with increased risk factors for coronary artery disease."

- John L. Ochsner, MD
Chairman Emeritus, Dept of Surgery
Ochsner Clinic, New Orleans, Louisiana
Past President (1989-91), International Society for Cardiovascular Surgery

"You Can Beat Heart Disease is a *wonderful resource* for heart patients and anyone interested in good health."

- Joseph C. Piscatella
Author, *Don't Eat Your Heart Out,* Tacoma, Washington

"Most other books in this field deal with a single factor -- for example, diet, exercise, smoking, weight, stress, or medications -- and describe how the action, absence, addition, and proper or improper use of this one factor will accelerate, slow down, prevent, or possibly even reverse the development of heart and artery disease. But experience has shown that correcting or modifying one factor is seldom effective in stopping heart disease.

"By contrast, Dr. Sauvage's new book tackles all of the many factors pertinent to the cause, prevention, and treatment of heart and artery diseases in a single, concise volume. By doing so he illuminates why all these factors must be marshalled into one powerful force to defeat cardiovascular disease, the greatest killer in the United States.

"Now that I have a book that tells me how to live a long and healthy life in clear words I can easily understand, I will use it to help my family and friends as well as myself. *This book is a true message of life,* and it will be my routine gift from this time on."

- John F. (Jack) Kiley
Recent coronary bypass patient, Olympia, Washington

"Dr. Sauvage's new *book* is an owner's manual for the human heart. Packed with useful information and helpful illustrations, it strips the confusion and mystery from the prevention of heart disease. At long last, here *is* the *user-friendly* resource that *belongs in every household.*"

- Nicholas J. Bez
Philanthropist, Seattle, Washington

"I really enjoyed reading this book. I must admit I find that most books for the lay public fail to strike a good balance between simplicity and enough information. This book is unique because it strikes that balance. In doing this, it gives a good idea about the underlying biology and discusses therapeutic approaches in a fair way that should be very helpful to patients trying to understand their physician's instructions."

- Stephen M. Schwartz, MD, PhD
Professor of Pathology
University of Washington School of Medicine, Seattle, Washington

"This is a *wonderful book* for my patients."

- J. Ward Kennedy, MD
Robert A. Bruce Professor of Medicine
University of Washington School of Medicine, Seattle, Washington

"This *timely monograph* provides an excellent balance of information regarding heart disease with equal attention to basic pathophysiology, practical patient efforts, and sophisticated medical interventions. As such, it will elicit broad interest from those who wish a comprehensive yet clear introduction to the prevention and treatment of heart disease. *I highly recommend this book."*

- Bradford C. Berk, MD, PhD
Professor of Medicine, Chief of Cardiology
Director of Cardiovascular Research
University of Rochester School of Medicine and Medical Center
Rochester, New York

"This book by a pioneer in the development of surgical techniques to treat heart disease is *particularly valuable* because it demonstrates how each of us can take control of our cardiovascular health status. Bravo, Dr. Sauvage!"

- Kaj H. Johansen, MD, PhD
Professor of Surgery, University of Washington School of Medicine
Seattle, Washington

"Dr. Sauvage and his collaborators have prepared an *unusually comprehensive basic* and factual treatise on the biology of the circulatory system with an emphasis on atherosclerosis and heart disease. Its engaging style and *highly understandable* language will make this *concise* book appealing to the vast audience of those who aren't schooled in the words of medicine. Many sections, such as the one detailing the essentials of an excellent program to abandon smoking, make it an especially useful guide to develop a heart-healthy lifestyle.

"Also impressive is Dr. Sauvage's understanding and clear delineation of the importance that an attitude of faith and hope plays in one's well-being."

- **Vallee L. Willman, MD**
Professor and Chairman Emeritus
St. Louis University School of Medicine, St. Louis, Missouri

"*You Can Beat Heart Disease* is an *essential book* for patients, families of patients, and physicians who have anything to do with taking care of patients with coronary or peripheral arterial disease. This concise, well-written text explains in accurate but simple terms the concepts of heart and artery diseases that are often misinterpreted and misevaluated by patients and physicians alike.

"This book is *invaluable* because it lets the readers understand that they have as much control over their own destiny as the physicians taking care of them. It instructs the patients on how to extend their longevity by modifying how they live their lives. I wholeheartedly recommend this book to anyone who intends to live over 50 years in the American culture."

- **R. Clement Darling III, MD**
Professor of Surgery
Chief, Division of Vascular Surgery
Director of Institute for Vascular Health and Disease
Albany Medical College, Albany, New York

"A *book* like this is *sorely needed,* so much so that I thought of doing one myself. Now that my good friend and colleague, Lester Sauvage, has done it so well, I can set this task aside. He has done us all a favor, and, as usual, *done it to perfection.*"

- **Robert B. Rutherford, MD**
Professor of Surgery Emeritus
University of Colorado, Denver, Colorado
Editor, Journal of Vascular Surgery

"Heart disease is *largely preventable*. In his book, *You Can Beat Heart Disease*, Dr. Sauvage and his team have clearly outlined the *principles* for us to *follow* to prolong our survival. **However, even a perfect lifestyle will not prevent the inevitable . . . we will all ultimately die.**

"Bodily well-being must not be our only goal. We also need to nourish and exercise our spiritual lives. We must decide what we believe about God, how we will relate to Him, and how our relationship with God will affect our interactions with others. That is why you must also read Dr. Sauvage's other book, *The Open Heart,* to complete the story. In it he describes how a life crisis can (and should) bring us closer to God. These two books, written by a surgeon who has held and healed many hearts, will help us to achieve both physical and spiritual health."

- H. Leon Greene, MD
Professor of Medicine, University of Washington
Author, *If I Should Wake Before I Die*
Seattle, Washington

"Besides being a skillful and caring surgeon, Dr. Sauvage is a talented writer. It is not common to see these two attributes together. His book *You Can Beat Heart Disease* is *concise, clear,* and *well organized.* Simple, but clear line drawings and half tone illustrations make it easy for the lay person to understand and enjoy the marvels of human biology, anatomy, and physiology.

"The most common diseases affecting the cardiovascular system are masterfully described in terms that everybody can understand. Their prevention and treatment are state of the art and a joy to read. Dr. Sauvage's book is full of common sense and sound advice that we must heed to live a quality life. A *fitting ending* to this wonderful book is the *Prayer of St. Francis.* The problems cursing our health care system today would be greatly lessened by remembering its closing words:

> '*For it is in giving that we receive,*
> *it is in pardoning that we are pardoned,*
> *and it is in dying*
> *that we are born to eternal life.'*"

- J. Leonel Villavicencio, MD
Professor of Surgery
Uniformed Services University of the Health Sciences, Bethesda, Maryland

Concluding Thoughts

Dr. H. Leon Greene, Author of *If I Should Wake Before I Die*, says in his endorsement on page 310, "You must also read Dr. Sauvage's other book, *The Open Heart,* to complete the story." I hope you will do this because these two books speak to the twin goals of achieving a long, healthy, and happy life here on earth, and then enjoying the infinitely greater happiness of Heaven for all eternity. In brief, these goals are **the essence of the how and the why to live.** They are, in fact, what real life is all about.

Writing the "whole" story for you has been a passion that grew within my soul as I performed open-heart surgery for 33 years. Having time to write these books after retiring from operative surgery has been a joy. I hope you will find them a source of good health, long life, and much happiness.*

Sincerely,

Lester R. Sauvage, MD,
Founder,
The Hope Heart Institute
528 18th Avenue
Seattle, WA 98122
206/903-2273
fax 206/903-2244
lsauvage@hopeheart.org
http://www.drsauvage.com

* If you have questions, please contact me, and I'll be happy to try and answer them for you.

Index

911 (Nine-one-one) 89,258,260
Adipocytes 150,286,287
Adipose tissue, 150,286,287
AICD (Automatic Internal Cardiac Defibrillator), 261-263
AIDS, 66
Alcohol, 54,152
Alveolus, 26,27
Amputation, leg, 117
Aneurysms, 4,5,72,77,82,83,108-111,115, 203,205,209,248,249,271
Angina Pectoris, 90,271
Angiogenesis, 298
Angioplasty (also see endovascular surgery), 93,206-215,217,231,240,243
    Abdomen, 233,235,240
    Carotids (brain), 229
    Coronaries (heart), 206-215,217
    Legs, 233-235,243
    Renals (kidneys), 230,231
Antibodies, 24
Anticoagulants, 271
Antioxidants, 197,271
Antioxidant Vitamins, 197
Antiplatelet medication, 198
Aorta, 5,58,108,271
Aortogram, 110,272
Apple shape, 186,286,290
Arrhythmia, 272
Arteries, 7,21,56,57,272
Arteriogram (Angiograms), 99,100,105-107
Arteriosclerosis, see Atherosclerosis
Aspirin, 198
Atherosclerosis,4-6,15,43,52,54,58,60,68,70,72-83,85,87-89,94,96,108,110,
    111,113-117,191,192,209,272,273,278,279, 284
Atherosclerosis and clotting, See Atherosclerosis
Automatic Internal Cardiac Defibrillator (AICD), 261-263
Better Life Diet, 112,136-160,191,193-195,199
Bile, 28
Blocked Arteries, 4-6,72-81,84-107, see bypass grafts, angioplasty, and stents
Blood, 64-67
Blood Clotting, 68-70,72-81, 272,273
Blood Pressure, 102,103,273
Body Mass Index (BMI), 151
Body Systems, 16-39
    Cardiovascular (heart, vessels, and blood), 20,21,44-83
    Digestive, 28,29
    Endocrine, 34,35
    Hematopoetic (blood cell forming), 22,23
    Integumentary (skin), 38,39
    Lymphatic/Immune, 24,25
    Musculoskeletal, 18
    Nervous, 19
    Reproductive, 36,37
    Respiratory, 26,27
    Urinary, 30-33
Bone marrow, 22,23
Boundary Organ Concept, 40-43
Brain attack, See Stroke
Butter, 140-142,282,283
Bypass Grafts, 202-204,216,218-227,232-239,244-247

Cancer, 24,25,66,115-118,123,273,274
Capillaries, 11,59,273,274
Carbohydrates, 40,137-141,143-147,150-160,193-195,274,283,284
Carbon Dioxide, 26,27,274
Carbon monoxide, 120,122-124
Cardiac Arrest and Ventricular Fibrillation, 42,258-260,275
Cardinal Rules (5) for Heart Healthy Living, 76,113,136,191-195
Cardiologist, 89-93,275
Cardiopulmonary Resuscitation (CPR), 258-260,275,276
CAT Scan, 110,111
Catheter, 92,202.207-209.280
Causes of Death, 5,88,272,273
Cell, 8-11
Cerebral Vascular Accident (Stroke -- Brain Attack), 94-101,276
Chlamydia Pneumoniae, 273
Cholesterol, 72,73,140,196,276,277
Chromosomes, 9,10
Clot dissolving drugs, 74,89
Clotting, *See* Blood Clotting
Coenzyme Q-10, 197
Collateral Circulation, 78-81,234,242,277
Collateral Vessels, 78-81,234,242,277
Common Carotid Artery, 94,95,277
Common Femoral Artery, 233-239,241,244-247,277
Common Iliac Artery, 108,240,277,278
Congestive heart failure, 54,55
Coronary Angioplasty (see *Angioplasty*)
Coronary Arteries, 52,53,278
Coronary Arteriograms, 86,92,93
Coronary Bypass Surgery, 212,213,216,218-223,226,227,278,297
Coronary Heart Disease, 73-75,88-93,278,279
Coronary Thrombosis, 278,279
Coumadin, 263,271
CPR (Cardiopulmonary Resuscitation), 258-260,275,276
Diabetes (type 1), 35,146,196,279,280
Diabetes (type 2), 35,113,115,138,143-146,151,196,279,280
Diagnosis of Aneurysms, 82,83,108-111
Diagnosis of Blocked Arteries, 84-107
    Brain, 94-101
    Heart, 88-93
    Kidneys, 102,103
    Legs, 104-107
Dialysis for kidney failure, 30,32,33
    Hemodialysis, 32,33
    Peritoneal Dialysis, 33
Diastole, 50
Diet, 76,113-115,136-160,190-195
Dietary Guidelines (7) of Better Life Diet, 138
DNA (Deoxyribonucleic acid), 8-10
Duplex (Doppler) Studies, 100,101
Echocardiogram, 90,91
Eggs, 138,146,154,156,157,195
Electrocardiogram, 85,91
Embolus, 70,71,94,96,98,276,280
Emphysema, 116,118,123,145
Endarterectomy, 203,204,229,241
Endothelium, 56,57,59,60
Endovascular Surgery (*also see* angioplasty), 93,206-215,217,231,240,280
ERT (Estrogen Replacement Therapy), 88,162,199,273
Erythropoietin, 30,102
Exercise, 76,113-115,141,161-187,192-194

Fats (Triglycerides), 4,40,72,73,137-160,192-196,276,277,281-283
    Monounsaturated, 281-283
    Polyunsaturated, 281-283
    Saturated, 72,153-160,281-283
Fiber, 72,137-141,143-145,150-160,283,284
Fibrin, 69
Fibrinogen, 69,115,120,193,196
Fish, 137-139,141,146,149,155,156,159,281,282,288
Flaxseed oil, 138,146,199,281,282
Food Groups, Five Basic, 145,146
Food Guide Block Diagram, 139,143
Foods high in saturated fats and *trans* fatty acids, 142
Free Radicals, 120,197,271
Gangrene, 106
Genes, 8,10,73,141,199
Gene Therapy, 242
Glossary, 271-290
Glucagon, 35,185,274
Gluconeogenesis, 288
Glucose, 35,140,144,150,185,274
Glycemic Index, 144,195,284
Glycogen, 35,144,150,185,274
Granulocytes, 64-67
Hardening of the arteries, *See* Atherosclerosis
HDL Cholesterol, 72,73,115,196,276
Healing cell, 298
Heart Attack, 4,88,89,284
Heart Failure (Congestive), 54,55
Heart-Healthy (Fit) Living, 76,112-199,209
    Five Cardinal Rules, 192-195
    Simple Plan, 190-199
    Three Additional Strategies, 196-199
Heart Scan, 86,90
Heart Transplantation, 264-266
Heart Valve Repair or Replacement, 224-227
Hemoglobin, 42,46,47,120,284,285
Hemorrhage, 94,285
Heparin, 271
High Blood Pressure, 4,115,285
HIV, 66
Homocysteine, 72,115,196,197,199
Hope Health Letter, 297
Hormones, 34,35
Immune System and Emaciation, 152
Infarct, 285
Inflammation, 65
Insulin, 35,115,141,144,150-152,274,279,280,285
Intermittent Claudication, 104,286
Internal Mammary Artery, 58,213,216,219,222,223,226
Ischemia, 286
Islets of pancreas, 34,35,274, 279,280,285
Isomer, 274,289
Kidney Failure, 4,30-33
LDL Cholesterol, 72,73,115,140,196,276,277
LDL Cholesterol Receptors, Inhibition of, 142,276,277,282,290
Legumes, 137-139,146,149,288
Life Cycle, 12-15
Lifestyle, 115,286
Lignan-rich flaxseed oil, 199,282
Lignans, 199
Limb loss, 115,117,138,144,163,191,193,196,286

Liposuction, 186
Liver, 28-29
Lose Excess Weight, 112-115,136-195,199
Lymphocytes, 64,65,66
Magnesium, 162,199
Margarine, 140-142,282,283
Meal Plan (7 day) and Nutritional Analysis for Better Life Diet, 153-160
Metabolism, 286
Milk, classification, 143
Monocytes/Macrophages, 64,65,67
MRI, 110
Murmur, 86,97,286
Muscles, 137,151,152,182,185,186,288
Myocardial Infarction, 89,285
Need for research, 297-299
Niacin, 141
Nicotine, 120,122-124
Nitric oxide, 174,176
Nutritional Basis for Better Life Diet©, 112-115,136-160,190-195
Obesity, 137,138,140,141,143-145,151,191,194,279,280,286
Off pump coronary bypass surgery, 213
Omega-3 & -6 essential fatty acids, 138,139,141,146,199,281,282
Omega-9 (oleic acid), 281
Open-Heart Surgery, 287
Ornish diet, 199
Osteoporosis, 88,118,162,173,199,287
Pacemakers, Artificial for the Heart, 254-257
Pacemaking and Conduction Systems of the Heart, 251-253
Peanut butter, 142,146,153,158,290
Pear shape, 186
Peripheral Vascular Disease, 287
Plaque, 287
        Hard, 4,73,75,272,273,287
        Lipid Core, 4,5,73,74,272,273,287
        Soft, 4,5,73,74,272,273,287
Plasma, 287
Platelet Aggregation, 67-71,73-75,198,272,273,287
Platelets, 22,23,64,65,67-71,73-75,198,272,273,287
Prayer of Saint Francis, 270
Prevention of Atherosclerosis, 76,112-199
        Dietary Information, 112-115,136-160,190-195,199
        Exercise, 112-115,161-187,190-194
        Smoking, 112-135,190-194
        Stress, 112-115,188,189,190-194
        Weight, 113-115,135-187,190-194
Primary Strategy to Beat Heart Disease, 1
Pritikin diet, 199
Proteins, 40,137-141,143,144,146,147,150-160,288
Providence Seattle Medical Center, xix
PTCA, 207,208,210,211,214,215,217,231,240,243
Pulse, 288,289
Red Blood Cells, 22,23,64,65
Renin, 86,102,103
Research, Need for, 297-299
Rest Pain, 104,105
Risk Factors for Heart Attack, 115,289
Risks and Consequences, 115
RNA (**Ribo**nucleic **a**cid), 10
Robotic coronary bypass surgery, 213
Salt, 199
Saphenous Vein, 61,213,218,220-222,227,245-247,289

Sauvage graft, 294
Selenium, 197
Shellfish, 137-139,141,149,288
SIDS, 116
Simple Plan for Heart-Healthy Living, 190-199
Sinus Node, 251-253
Smoking, 112-135,190-194
Spiritual Reflections, 267-270
Starvation, 152,288
"Statin drugs," 141,197
Stents, 208,209,211,212,215,217,230,231,233,234,240,243
Stethoscope, 86,97
Stress, 112-115,188,189
Stroke, 4,94-101
Sudden cardiac death, 115,258-260,275
Sugar, 72,115,136-141,143-145,150-160,193-195,274,284,289,290
Surgery for Aneuryms, 203,205,209,248,249
Surgery to Increase the Blood Supply, 200-241,243-247
　　　to the Brain, 228,229
　　　to the Heart, 212-227
　　　to the Kidneys, 230-232
　　　to the Legs, 233-241,243-247
Surgical Procedures, 200-241,243-249,254-257,261-266
　　　Endovascular,200,201,206-215,217,230,231,233-235, 240,243
　　　Vascular, 200-205,212,213,216,218-230,232-239,241,244-249
Swedish Medical Center, xix
Syndrome X, 150,290
Systole, 51
Tar, 122,123
Thrombopoietin, 67
Thrill, 86
TIA, 71,98-101
Trans Fatty Acids,72,115,136-143,145,148,149,153-160,193,195,276,277,282,290
Transplantation - Heart, 264-266
Transplantation - Kidney, 30
Treadmill, 85,91,92
Triglycerides (Fats), 4,40,72,73,137-160,192-196,276,277,281-283
Turbulence, 86,97
Twenty ways to lower saturated fat and *trans* fatty acid in diet, 148,149
Two Main Complications of Atherosclerosis, 4-6,72-83
Ultrasound Studies, 86,100-102,110
　　　Aorta, 110
　　　Carotids,100,101
　　　Kidneys, 102
　　　Legs, 86
Valves of Heart, 48-51
Valves of Veins, 60,62,63
Vascular Surgery, 202-205 (also see Surgical Procedures, Vascular)
Veins, 60-63,290
Ventricular fibrillation and cardiac arrest, 258-260,275,276
Weight Control:
　　　Basics for. 150-152,288
　　　Gain when too thin, 152,288
　　　Lose excess, 112-115,136-195,199
　　　Maintain ideal weight, 151
White Blood Cells (Granulocytes, lymphocytes, and monocytes),
　　　22,23,64-67
Women and heart diease, 5,88,90,116,117, 199,273
Zyban, 128